Run Fast. Eat Slow.

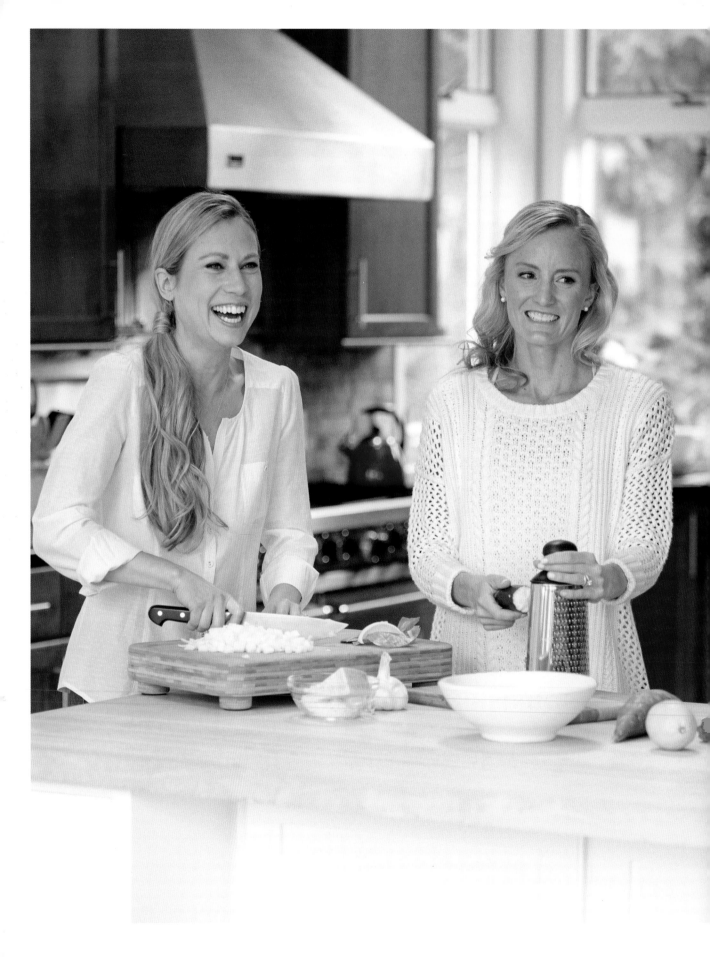

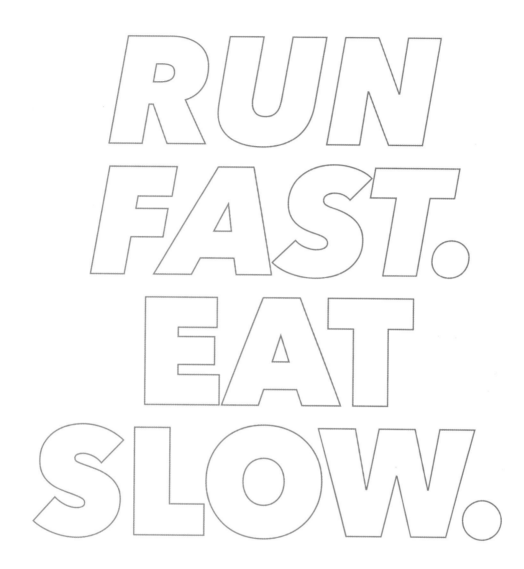

RUN FAST. EAT SLOW.

NOURISHING RECIPES FOR ATHLETES

Shalane Flanagan and Elyse Kopecky

Photography by Alan Weiner

RODALE.

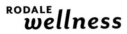

RODALE *wellness*

Live happy. Be healthy. Get inspired.

Sign up today to get exclusive access to our authors, exclusive bonuses,
and the most authoritative, useful, and cutting-edge information on health,
wellness, fitness, and living your life to the fullest.

Visit us online at RodaleWellness.com
Join us at RodaleWellness.com/Join

Rodale books may be purchased for business or promotional use or for special sales. For information, please write to:
Special Markets Department, Rodale Inc., 733 Third Avenue, New York, NY 10017.

Printed in China

Rodale Inc. makes every effort to use acid-free ∞, recycled paper ♻.

Book design by Christina Gaugler

Cover design by Tad Greenough and Sezay Altinok

Photographs by Alan Weiner, with the exception of the following: Victor Sailer/PhotoRun, xiii; Carlos Serrao, xiv, 206;
Nike Running, 47 (*bottom right*); Andy Hughes, 47 (*top*); the authors, 47 (*bottom left*), 93, 226 (*childhood photo*),
and 227 (*childhood photo*)

Library of Congress Cataloging-in-Publication Data is on file with the publisher.

ISBN-13: 978-1-62336-681-0

Distributed to the trade by Macmillan

11   hardcover

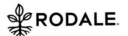

RODALE.

We inspire and enable people to improve their lives and the world around them.

For my training partners and teammates
who added inspiration, richness, motivation,
and giggles to my running adventure
—SF

For my three loves: Lily for showing me pure joy,
Andy for washing endless dishes,
and Huckleberry for licking all the spills off the ground
—EK

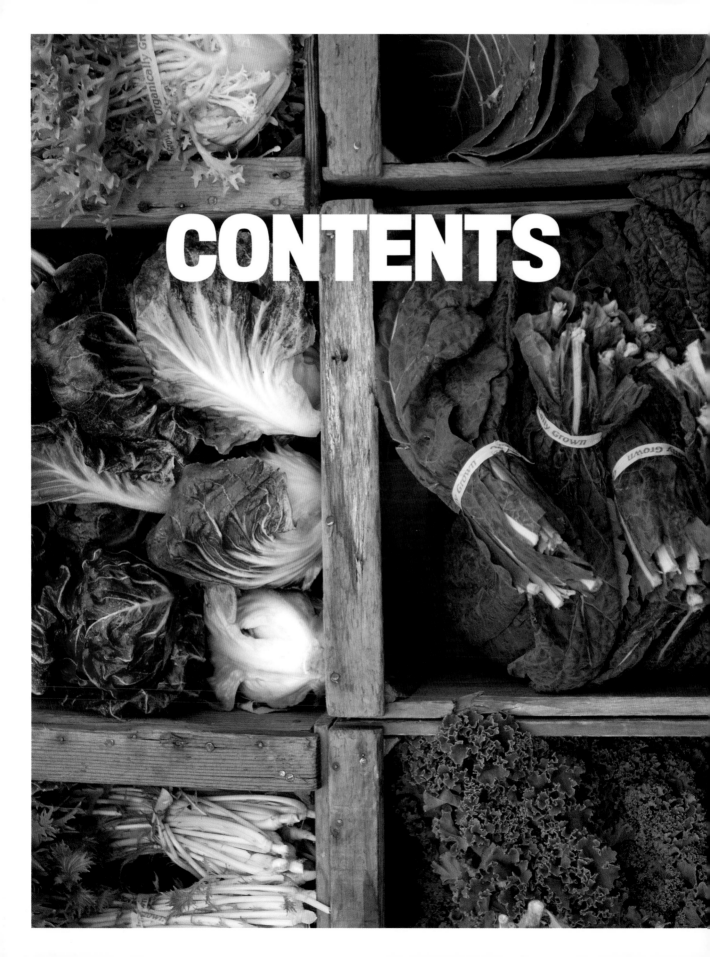

CONTENTS

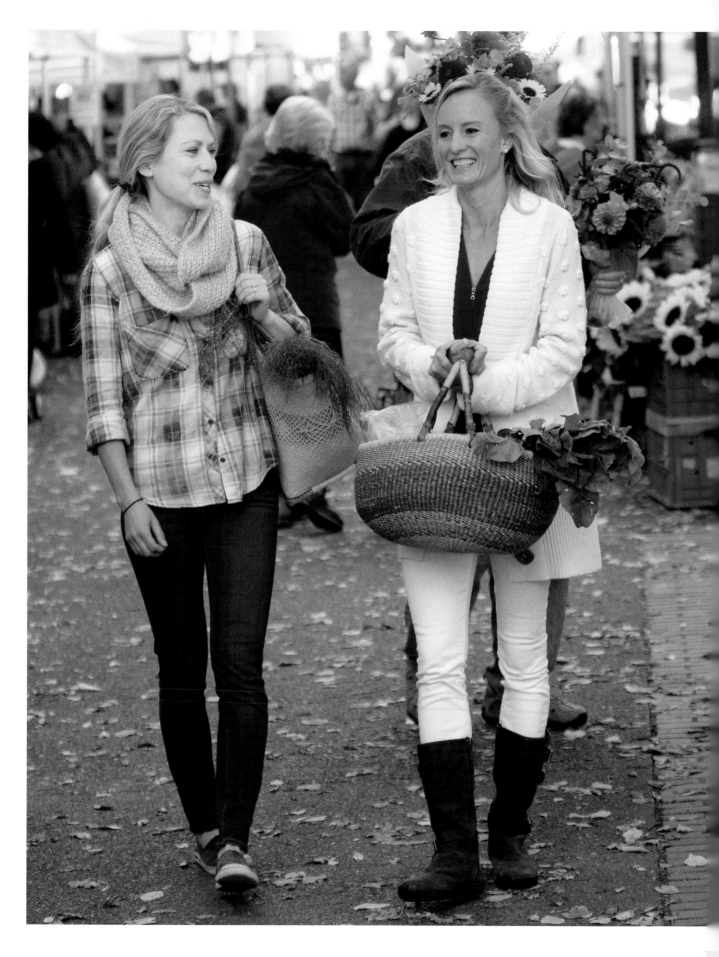

Introduction

I knocked, and Steve, Shalane's husband, answered the door. Shalane was manning the grill on the back deck of her home high up in the southwestern hills of Portland. It was one of those flawless end-of-summer evenings that begs for catching up with old friends. I thought about how much Shalane had accomplished since we were anxious freshmen on the cross-country team at the University of North Carolina. I wondered if I would even be able to keep up with her for 1 mile at her marathon pace.

I made a beeline for the patio, and we shrieked in excitement and embraced. The last time we had seen each other was more than 2 years ago in NYC for Shalane's memorable marathon debut. I was working for Nike Running at the time, and Shalane was running for Nike. After graduation we had both moved west to Portland, so our paths had stayed very much intertwined, until I moved abroad.

"It's been forever," Shalane said. "I want to hear everything about your life in Switzerland. And I can't believe you quit your job to go to culinary school in NYC. How was it?"

"Seriously, we have so much to catch up on. But you go first, because I've been watching all your races from afar and want to hear firsthand how you do it. I still get goose bumps every time I watch you run 26.2 against the best in the world!" I exclaimed.

"Wait, let me get you a drink. What did you bring? That salad looks phenomenal. What's in it?"

"You'll have dreams about it after I leave here," I joked. "It's a kale-radicchio salad with farro and my signature lemon miso dressing. I could drink this dressing. It's addicting."

Our conversation continued at three times the normal pace (think *Shalane-fast*) and jumped back and forth between catching up on our lives, random memories from college, and exclamations on how much I had missed Portland—especially the local food scene, the farmers' market, and the endless running trails. Our husbands elected to hover inside with their microbrews while we flipped the burgers on the grill, chattered like teenagers on too much caffeine, and enjoyed the swoon-worthy view of Mount Hood.

We reminisced about the dishes we cooked when we lived together in college, including our meat fondue party that left everyone racing for the toilet. At least we *attempted* to cook back then. So many of our teammates lived off of cold cereal, protein bars, and Pop-Tarts slathered with peanut butter. I shared with Shalane how,

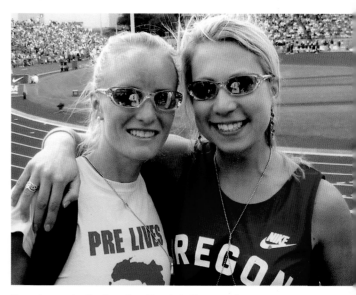

Together at the Prefontaine Classic in Eugene, Oregon, June 2005

even after graduating from culinary school, I still considered her famous Breakfast-Meets-Dinner rice bowl a regular part of my comfort-food repertoire.

We moved inside to the dining table and dug in to an enticing spread of juicy bison burgers, cumin-spiced sweet potato fries, and my show-stopping salad. I excitedly started to fill Shalane in on everything I had been studying about food and nutrition and its life-changing impact on my health and happiness—and how it could help Shalane in pursuit of her fourth Olympic team.

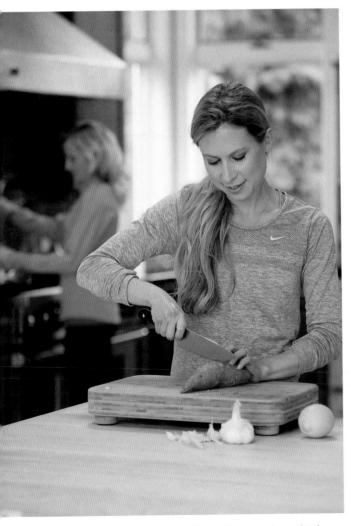

Elyse making sweet potato fries in Shalane's home kitchen.

We talked about the misconceptions around what constitutes healthy eating and how the alarming diet trends and endless health-claiming food products were doing more harm than good.

"What if people knew how well we eat? I think they'd be alarmed by how much olive oil and butter I go through in a week," Shalane said.

"The perception is that healthy food is bland, boring, and uncool," I said. "The reality is it can be delicious and incredibly satisfying. Our friends are seriously missing out."

The simple, seasonal dishes shared between longtime friends inspired the conversation at the table that night. Shalane shared her concerns about her own diet and her realization that as she gets older, she can't get away with lackluster nutrition, especially with training 120 miles a week. I shared my dreams of starting a family soon and how switching to a whole foods diet rich in good fats helped me overcome a 15-year battle with athletic amenorrhea, the absence of menstruation.

We talked about how female runners in this country are experiencing infertility rates at an all-time high. I shared my belief that a huge part of the problem is that women aren't getting enough nourishing fats in their diets. "We still have a fear of fat in this country," I said. "I realized this when I moved abroad to Switzerland and saw the difference in the food. The whole milk yogurt there was rich, creamy, and pure, not stripped of fat and flavor with added sugar, artificial flavoring, and a measly strawberry to make up for it."

We shared ideas and thought: What if we wrote a book for athletes unlike any of the "light and lean" running cookbooks out there. Our book would celebrate all whole foods instead of obsessing over carbs verses protein or the latest diet trend? We would show runners everywhere that by indulging—yes, *indulging*—in real food,

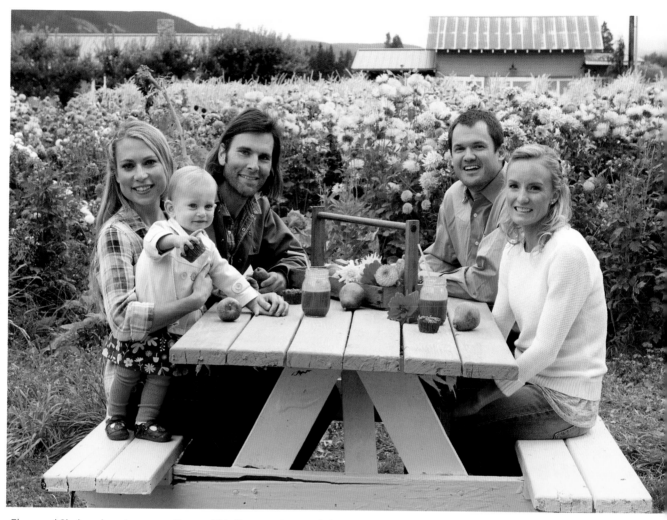

Elyse and Shalane hanging out at Draper Girls Country Farm with their husbands, Andy and Steve, and Elyse's daughter, Lily.

they will not only train and perform better, but also improve their overall health, all while enjoying what they eat more than ever before.

And so—over that nourishing, home-cooked summer meal at Shalane's home—it was decided. *Run Fast Eat Slow* had been born.

After dinner, Shalane took me on a tour of her house to see all the renovations they had made recently. For a world-class runner with a long list of accomplishments, her polished, white-walled home was surprisingly free of any running para-phernalia. Even her cherished medal from the

Beijing Olympics was nowhere to be seen. When I asked where she kept her bronze beauty, she explained nonchalantly that she keeps it tucked away in her sock drawer in order to not get complacent.

To kick off our cookbook project, Shalane kept a food journal leading up to the Berlin Marathon in which she recorded the foods she ate to maximize her performance. After that we spent hours together in my kitchen developing her favorite foods into crave-worthy, approach-able recipes.

After a racing season spent devouring the nourishing recipes we were developing for this book, Shalane found that her racing weight came naturally—no deprivation needed. She was enjoying food more than ever and was recovering faster from her grueling 24-mile training runs at 6,910 feet. Shalane went on to run a personal record in the marathon in her hometown of Boston, set the 10-K American road record, and qualified for her fourth Olympic team in the marathon. And Elyse went on to writing this book full-time shortly after becoming an overjoyed mom of a healthy baby girl.

Each recipe in *Run Fast Eat Slow* was carefully crafted—using Shalane as the guinea pig—to maximize flavor and nutrition (luckily the two can go hand in hand) and to minimize inflammation, digestive distress, and toxins. The whole foods, flavor-forward recipes are approachable for the beginner cook, simple for the time-starved, inspiring for skilled chefs, and nourishing for anyone living an active life.

Once we perfected more than 100 of our

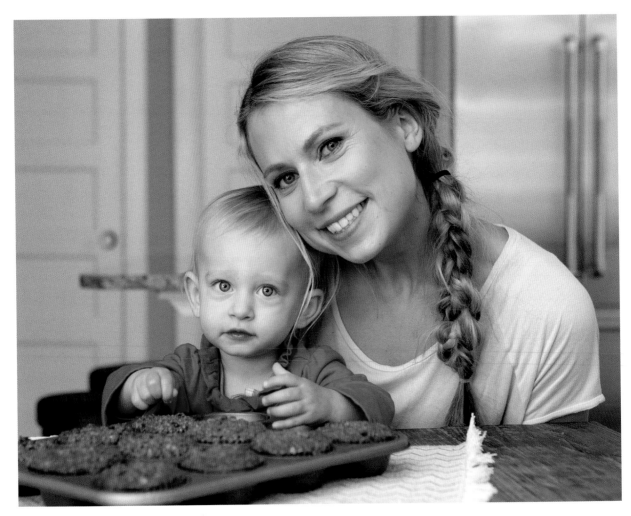

Elyse sharing Superhero Muffins with her daughter, Lily.

INTRODUCTION

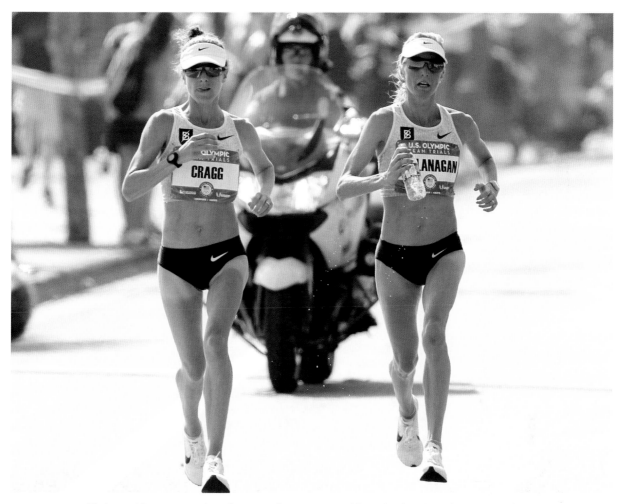

Shalane with teammate Amy Cragg on their way to qualifying for the 2016 Olympic Marathon.

favorite recipes, we sent them out to be vetted by an incredible team of runners. The team included a high school cross-country runner with aspirations to run in college, an elite marathoner training for the Rio Olympics, an ultramarathoner-CEO, a PhD physicist, a running store owner, a breast cancer oncologist, and even a dad inspired to cook healthier for his active family (shout-out to our dedicated team of hungry testers!). We also had the recipes professionally tested by the lovely Megan Scott from *Joy of*

Cooking. Best of all, Shalane, despite her crazy training and travel schedule, road-tested every single recipe in this book.

Recipe testing is long over, but we continue to cook from our own book—because this is the food we love to eat and love to share with our friends and family. And now we're beyond thrilled to share this collection of our best recipes and mind-blowing nutritional wisdom with you. Get ready to chop, sauté, simmer, and bake your way to your next PR!

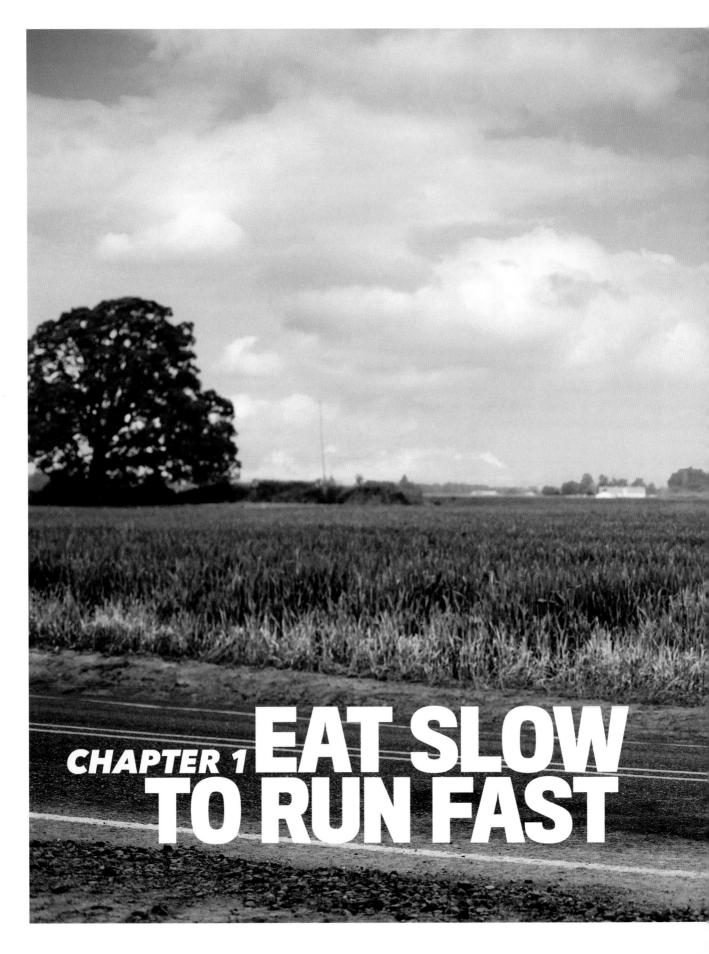

CHAPTER 1 **EAT SLOW TO RUN FAST**

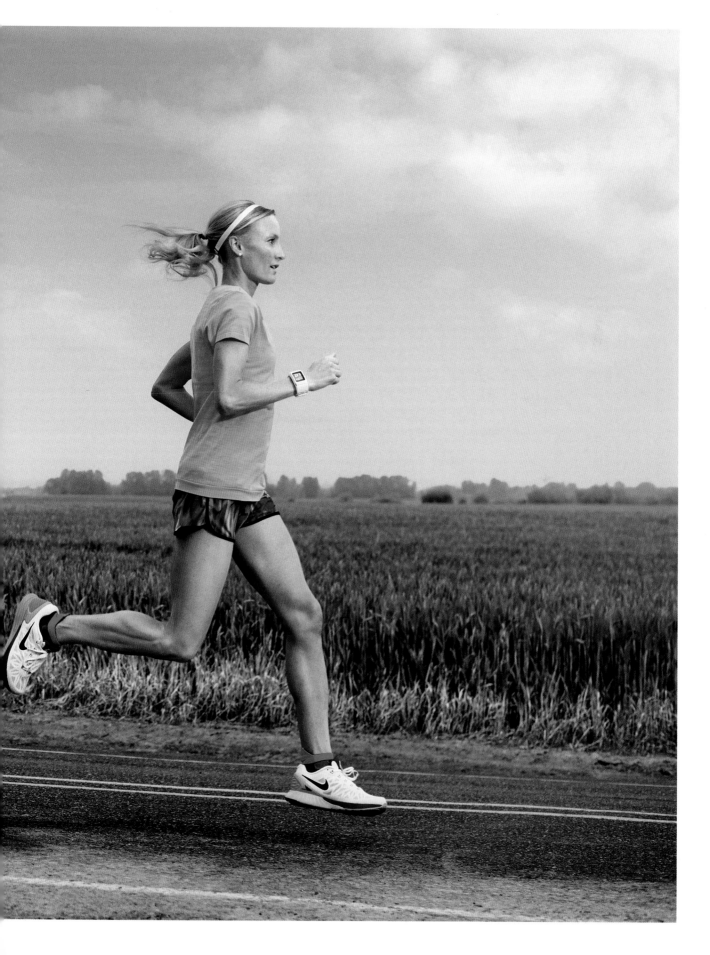

As runners we are so focused on our immediate energy needs that we obsess over macronutrients and forget that not all proteins, fats, and carbs are created equal. The stress that running puts on the body means that to stay healthy, runners need more antioxidants, vitamins, and minerals than most. In a culture accustomed to processed foods, produce shipped from halfway around the world, and factory-farmed meats, it's more difficult than ever to fulfill our nutritional needs. As a result, runners everywhere are missing out on the nourishment their bodies need to thrive.

The chance to teach endurance athletes like you how to nourish your body for the long run is what inspired us to pour our hearts into this book. We aren't suggesting you eat this way solely to crush your PR or to cross the finish line first. This book can help you do just that, but we're also looking past the finish line and aiming for lifelong health and happiness.

Before you dive into our recipes, we want to impart some of our healthy-eating wisdom. For us, deciding what to eat, in order to eat well, has become second nature—a way of life. But to many of our fellow runners, our way of eating might at first sound foreign and daunting. Fear not. You're about to discover that our approach to maximizing nourishment so that your body can perform at its best puts flavor and fun at the forefront.

We all know what "run fast" means, right? Get out there and kick some @#*! We want you to be able to do just that and more. In a broader sense, "run fast" means not just surviving but thriving in our insanely fast-paced lifestyles—lifestyles that don't seem conducive to having the time (or energy) to cook. We'll convince you otherwise!

But what do we really mean by "eat slow"? It means so much more than simply taking the time to chew your food. It represents our way of eating that includes preparing nourishing meals from scratch, sitting down at a table instead of eating on the go, enjoying food in the company of friends and family, seeking out foods that were grown or raised with care, and tuning in to what our bodies need to thrive.

RUNNING ON EMPTY

Despite all the medical discoveries over the last 50 years, humankind is far from thriving. In fact, we are less healthy today than our grandparents. For the first time in history, children born today potentially have a shorter life expectancy than their parents. Occurrences of chronic diseases like cancer, heart disease, diabetes, and depression are at an all-time high. Studies show that unhealthy diets are a leading cause of these preventable diseases.

Although runners are put on a pedestal as the epitome of health, we know all too well that runners and other endurance athletes are far from immune to these serious health issues. The convenience foods coveted by runners, including bars, gels, and sports drinks, not only lack real nutrition, but also are high in inflammatory foods like refined grains, processed sweeteners, industrial oils, and artificial ingredients.

There are more than 600,000 food items in the marketplace today: 80 percent of them have added sugar, and the majority of packaged foods are nutrient poor and contain chemical additives. Scary, considering that for most Americans, packaged foods make up 70 percent of their diet.

As a result of our reliance on nutrient-poor processed foods, the majority of Americans are overfed, undernourished, and running on empty. Refined foods provide mass without sustenance. For an athlete, running on empty can lead to immediate negative consequences and long-term health concerns.

On top of this, runners are constantly bombarded with messages about weight loss, calorie counts, juice cleanses, low-carb diets, low-fat diets—the list goes on. These messages lead to an unhealthy relationship with food, imbalanced eating, food phobias, obsessions over weight loss, yo-yo dieting, cravings, undernourishment, weight fluctuations, and eating disorders.

It is estimated that at least half of the running population is sidelined at some point during the year due to an injury. The right nourishment can help an athlete recover from injury. Food can be incredibly healing, but the Standard American Diet (SAD) is high in inflammatory foods and low in healing foods. For an athlete who is constantly breaking down the body during intense training sessions, nutrient-dense foods are critical to a faster recovery time.

According to Ron Thompson, PhD, FAED, CEDS, coauthor of *Eating Disorders in Sport*, "When coaches and athletes are asked what is the major contributor to good athletic performance, they often say things like VO$_2$ max, training load, or a particular type of training. Such factors are important in sport performance, but with such responses, athletes and coaches are missing the basics. Other than genetics, the major contributor to good athletic performance is good health, and the major contributor to good health (other than genetics) is good nutrition. The well-nourished athlete will not only perform better, but will perform better longer."

With so much misleading information out there—most of it driven by food corporations—it's no surprise that something as basic and intuitive as eating has become so complex. The result of being bombarded with food products everywhere we turn is that we're no longer in tune with one of our most basic needs: eating. We have lost the instinct to reach for the foods that will best fuel our demanding lifestyles.

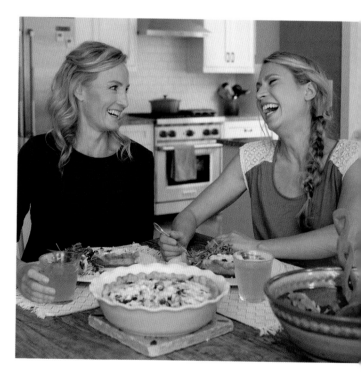

INDULGENT NOURISHMENT

"Indulgent nourishment" is how we define our way of eating. We know our hardworking bodies need substantial fuel, so we indulge in our favorite whole foods. By filling up on the healthful foods we love and not obsessing over calorie counts, carbs, or fat, we're able to eat in tune with what our bodies need. We know that real food leads to serious satisfaction and allows the body to function optimally without weight gain.

On the other hand, we believe that dieting leads to imbalanced eating, which results in sugar cravings, snack attacks, and, in the end, weight gain. Instead of focusing on calorie counts, we focus our energy on eating a balanced diet rich in wholesome foods—foods that keep us energized and satisfied.

The recipes in this cookbook do not include calorie counts or macronutrient (carbs, protein, fat) measurements. This wasn't an oversight but intentional. Don't ask us how many grams of protein are in our High-Altitude Bison Meatballs with Simple Marinara (page 120) or how many grams of fat are in our Superhero Muffins (page 42). We don't know and we don't care. Instead we'll tell you all about the incredible phytochemicals, antioxidants, and omega 3s and the exciting ways these delicious foods can help supercharge your training.

All macronutrients are not created equal. Judging the health of a food based on how many grams of protein or fat it has is dangerous because these numbers don't reveal the nutrient quality of the food. It's akin to buying a pair of running shoes based solely on their weight without looking at the quality of the technology or considering how the shoe feels on your foot.

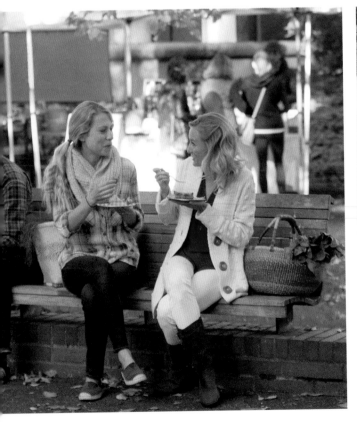

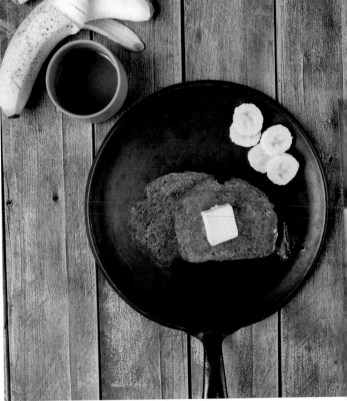

EATING REAL FOOD

When deciding what to eat to eat well, it's best to look at the full picture, including where the food came from, how it was grown, how much it was processed, how it tastes, and, most important, how it makes you feel.

For us that means eating a varied diet that includes meat, veggies, fruit, cultured dairy, legumes, whole grains, nuts, seeds, and more. We avoid processed foods and limit our consumption of refined grains and sugar—these foods don't make us feel good. We seek out organic and local ingredients as much as possible and enjoy eating with the seasons, since food picked at its peak not only tastes better, but also is more nutrient dense.

We don't eat meat every single day, but we do believe it is healthy to include on a regular basis in our diets. In many of our dishes, the veggies shine and meat becomes the loyal side companion. As much as possible, we try to get our meat from trusted local farmers who care about the planet. The free-range chicken, beef, bison, and lamb we buy is expensive, but our philosophy is to eat better quality meat and less of it for maximum nourishment.

Not everyone can afford to buy organic all the time, but when possible try to stick to organic, local, or sustainable options when it comes to meat, seafood, dairy, and the produce on the Environmental Working Group's "Dirty Dozen" list (annual list of the most pesticide-ridden produce). Consider ways to make budget cuts elsewhere to make good food a priority. In the United States, we spend less on food than any other developed country, a mere 6.4 percent of our total spending, and we spend more than

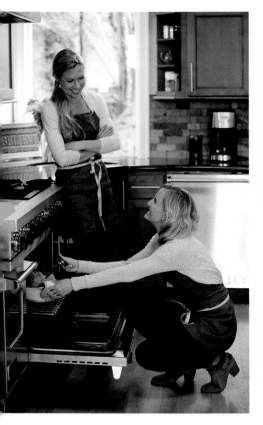

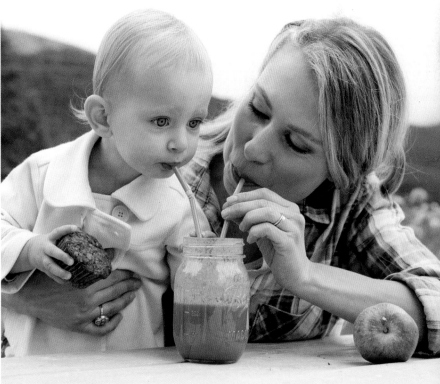

any other country on health care. Spending at the grocery store or farmers' market is an investment in your future.

We hope you'll find this to be a refreshing way to eat. If you're eating mostly whole foods, you don't need numbers to eat healthy and balanced. But it might be difficult to let go of the numbers at first and get in tune with your body's hunger signals. In our society, we're programmed to think of food in terms of calories or cost (negatives) instead of in terms of nourishment and satisfaction (positives). Slowing down, taking the time to cook, and enjoying every bite will help.

FAT FOR FLAVOR AND FUEL

In our recipes, we make no apologies for the amount of fat. We sauté with olive oil, bake with butter and coconut oil, stir in whole milk yogurt, simmer with coconut milk, and drizzle on dressings and sauces.

Why?

Fat is a carrier for flavor and nutrients. Many vitamins and minerals cannot be absorbed without it. Fat is also a primary source of energy—viable energy that can fuel your body for endurance endeavors. A meal rich in healthy fats will leave you feeling satisfied, better nourished, and less likely to reach for a sugar fix.

Runners often obsess over carbohydrates and protein and forget that fat is also an important building block. Both saturated and unsaturated fat from whole foods is critical for healthy brain function, cardiovascular strength, hormone balance, building lean muscle, and combating inflammation. Studies show a diet rich in good fats actually boosts metabolism instead of causing weight gain.

Female athletes in particular can suffer hormone imbalances without enough fat in their diets. It's estimated that 20 percent of active women and up to 45 percent of female competitive runners suffer from athletic amenorrhea, which can lead to bone loss and fertility issues. When the body isn't getting enough fuel, it begins to shut down systems that aren't necessary for survival, and the female reproductive system is one of the first to go. Getting more high-quality calories in the diet can reverse this detrimental condition.

The fats we love for their health-giving properties and ability to transform the mundane into magic include nuts, seeds, avocados, coconut oil, olive oil, whole milk yogurt, meat, and butter (learn more about these fats in Chapter 2).

On the other hand, the oils found in packaged and fast foods are often unhealthy hydrogenated fats made in a lab via a harsh chemical process to give them a long shelf life. These inflammatory fats don't have any health-redeeming properties and are stored by the body instead of burned as fuel, leading to weight gain and an increased risk of heart disease. Not cool.

We've been programmed to think of fat as bad, but remember that not all are created equal. The fats we use in the recipes that follow are body-loving, nutrient-dense, energizing fats.

Health food unfortunately has gotten a bad rap over the years for being bland and boring. It doesn't have to be. There's a wealth of nutrients in a range of your favorite foods (and no, they're not just vegetables!) that you'll be thrilled to discover in Chapter 2 as we take you on a tour of our pantries.

EAT LIKE SHALANE

Without measuring calories, you might wonder how Shalane achieves her optimal race weight. Shalane does make a conscious effort every single day to eat fresh, whole foods, but she doesn't follow a diet plan. She would rather save her mad math skills for counting miles and calculating splits. She avoids processed foods and sugary snacks because these foods provide little sustenance and displace the real foods her body craves.

Leading up to a big race, Shalane will limit her consumption of sweets and give up her occasional glass of wine. Otherwise she eats like she always eats—with an appetite for nourishment and an appreciation for good food.

Since Shalane started devouring the recipes in this book, her ideal racing weight now comes naturally, without deprivation. She no longer craves sugary snacks, and she feels satisfied after every meal. This has been a refreshing game changer, allowing her to have fun in the kitchen. She now views cooking as a training tool that's as important as her next workout.

To help you make the transition to a balanced whole foods–based diet, we've provided an outline of what a typical week of eating looks like for Shalane. We've included cross-references to the recipes in this book that she can't live without. We've also listed her go-to recipes for fueling for race day, including what she eats the night before and the morning of her big marathons.

It's important to remember that different foods affect everyone differently. You should always listen to your own body and eat what makes you feel good. Never try anything new the night before or on race day. Practice eating new foods before your training runs and learn what you digest best.

MARATHON-READY FAVORITES

Prerace Dinner

Flu-Fighter Chicken and Rice Stew, page 108

High-Altitude Bison Meatballs with Simple Marinara, page 120

Wild Salmon Sweet Potato Cakes, page 142

Parmesan and Herb-Crusted Cod, page 150

Sweet Potato Fries, page 161

Marathon Day Breakfast

Race Day Oatmeal (with banana, nuts, raisins), page 53

Toast with homemade nut butter (Sweet Cinnamon Tahini Butter, page 204, or Coffee-Vanilla Peanut Butter, page 205)

Coffee

Hydration drink

Postrace Celebration

Don't Get Beet Hummus, page 73, with Pita Chips with Oregano and Sea Salt, page 74

Greek Bison Burgers, page 138, with Avocado Cream, page 178

Oregon microbrew

Doughnuts . . . shh, don't tell

Flourless Almond Torte, page 184

Eat Like Shalane

	MONDAY	TUESDAY	WEDNESDAY
Breakfast	Coffee Water Scrambled eggs with spinach Whole grain toast with butter Can't Beet Me Smoothie (page 28)	Coffee Water Swiss Muesli Bowl (page 46) with berries Banana	Coffee Water Race Day Oatmeal (page 53) Sweet Potato Breakfast Cookie (page 56)
Lunch	Kale-Radicchio Salad with Farro (page 80) Apple with nut or seed butter (Sweet Cinnamon Tahini Butter, page 204, or Coffee-Vanilla Peanut Butter, page 205)	Leftover Recovery Quinoa Salad (page 99), topped with a hard-boiled egg	Leftover Wild West Rice Salad (page 90) Leftover salmon Dark chocolate
Snack	Energizing Chai (page 38) Superhero Muffin (page 42)	Whole milk yogurt with Ginger-Molasses Granola (page 54) Banana	26.2 Trail Mix (page 62) Coconut-Kale Smoothie (page 31)
Dinner	Crostini with Arugula Cashew Pesto (page 68) Recovery Quinoa Salad (page 99) Grilled steak	Fish Tacos with Mango-Avocado Salsa (page 136) Wild West Rice Salad (page 90)	High-Altitude Bison Meatballs with Simple Marinara (page 120) Arugula salad with roasted veggies and Basic Balsamic Vinaigrette (page 169)
Dessert	Double Chocolate Teff Cookie (page 187) Herbal tea	Cocoa-Coconut Macaroons (page 196) Herbal tea	Apple slices with nut or seed butter (Sweet Cinnamon Tahini Butter, page 204, or Coffee-Vanilla Peanut Butter, page 205) Herbal tea

In a typical week, Shalane will bake one or two wholesome treats for snacks and dessert and rely on leftovers more often. The above includes more variety to showcase all her favorites.

THURSDAY	FRIDAY	SATURDAY	SUNDAY
Coffee Water Superhero Muffin (page 42) Banana and berries	Coffee Water Teff Pumpkin Pancakes with Currants (page 44) Can't Beet Me Smoothie (page 28)	Coffee Water Whole grain toast with Sweet Cinnamon Tahini Butter (page 204) Banana	Coffee Water Whole milk yogurt with Ginger-Molasses Granola (page 54) and berries
Root Lovers' Winter Salad (page 84) Don't Get Beet Hummus (page 73) with Pita Chips with Oregano and Sea Salt (page 74)	Omega Sardine Salad (page 94) on whole grain bread	Leftover Moroccan Lentil Salad with Cauliflower Couscous (page 96) topped with leftover chicken	Sandwich made with leftover chicken and sliced avocado Broccoli Chèvre Soup (page 102)
26.2 Trail Mix (page 62) Runner's Recovery Iced Tea (page 36)	Banana slathered with Coffee-Vanilla Peanut Butter (page 205) Energizing Chai (page 38)	Half avocado with Dulse Mineral Salt (page 179) Giddy-Up Energy Bites (page 57) Green tea	Spelt Banana Bread (page 183) Energizing Chai (page 38)
Soba Noodle Salad with Runner's High Peanut Sauce (page 87)	Moroccan Lentil Salad with Cauliflower Couscous (page 96) Whole Roasted Chicken with Herbs (page 130)	Carrot-Ginger Soup (page 116) Zucchini Quinotto with Roasted Garlic (page 145)	Shalane's Breakfast-Meets-Dinner Bowl (page 128) with Avocado Cream (page 178)
Flourless Almond Torte (page 184) Herbal tea	Dates and dried apricots Runner's Recovery Iced Tea (page 36)	Ginger-Molasses Quick Bread (page 186) Apple-Ginger Cider (page 39)	Pecan Butter Chocolate Truffles with Sea Salt (page 191) Herbal tea

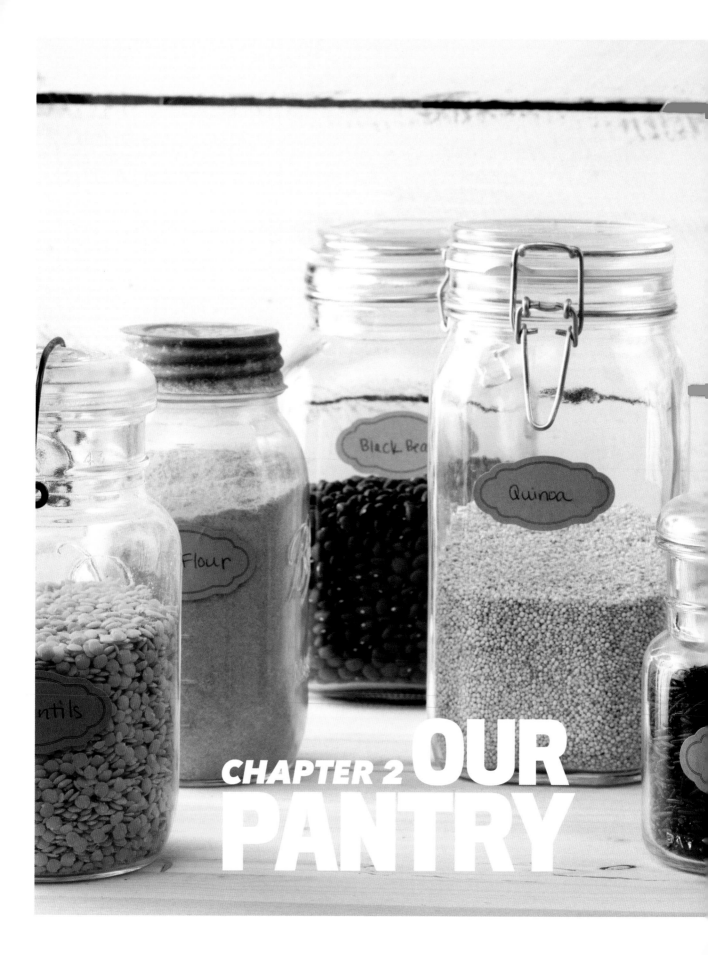

CHAPTER 2 OUR
PANTRY

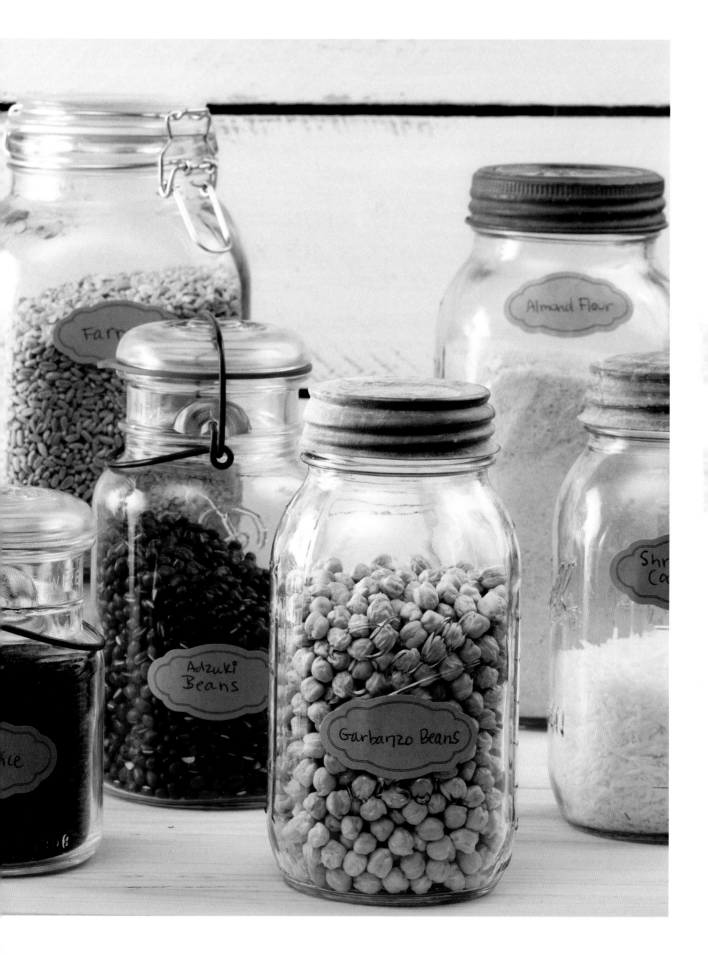

The biggest obstacle to cooking fresh food on a daily basis is a poorly stocked kitchen. When you're squeezing in a run after class or work and your stomach begins grumbling on the drive home, takeout sounds way more enticing than waiting in line at the grocery store. With a well-stocked pantry and a few staples waiting in your fridge, there will always be something delicious that you can get on the table fast.

In this chapter, we'll take you on a tour of our kitchens. Come peer into our pantries and fridges to see the ingredients that we always keep on hand. These are the foods that fuel Shalane's demanding training regimen and Elyse's hectic working-momma schedule. By stocking these ingredients, you'll be well prepared to cook all the incredible recipes in this book. A recipe is much less daunting when you only need to run out for a few fresh ingredients.

Another benefit of keeping a stocked pantry is that when you do hit the grocery store, you can stick to the perimeter and avoid the endless aisles of processed foods. Or better yet, avoid the grocery store and hit up a farmers' market on a weekly basis to pick up fresh favorites.

What follows is an alphabetical list of the ingredients you'll want to stock to power your athletic endeavors—whether that's training for a marathon or chasing after a toddler. With each, we've included a few nutrition fun facts, culinary tips, storage tips, and more. Most of our power foods have too much of a good thing to list all the benefits in a short paragraph. Therefore, if you're interested in learning more, flip to our Resources section (page 220).

We've divided the following list into Pantry Staples, Fridge Staples, and Fresh Favorites. Ready to stock up on wholesome basics? Here we go.

PANTRY STAPLES

BAKING BASICS

To fuel our baking addiction, we keep a few key ingredients on hand such as unsweetened cocoa powder, vanilla and almond extracts, baking powder, baking soda, and of course, dark chocolate.

Usually the dark chocolate never makes it into our recipes since we end up snacking on it! Lucky for us (and you!) we con-sider chocolate to be a super-food. Just look for a bar that has a 70% or higher cocoa content. Dark chocolate (sorry, not milk) is full of antioxidants, vitamins, and minerals. We find that a square of dark chocolate after breakfast (Elyse) or lunch (Sha-lane) curbs sweet cravings for the rest of the day.

When buying baking powder, look for a brand that is free of aluminum. For almond and vanilla extracts, check the labels and avoid brands with artificial flavorings.

BROTH

We keep boxed low-sodium chicken and vegetable broths stocked in our pantries and homemade broth stocked in our freezers. When buying broth, seek out an organic brand to avoid any additives and check the label to find one without sugar added. With broth on hand, you can turn out a nourishing soup or stew in under 30 minutes simply by simmering together any assortment of vegetables, beans, and whole grains.

Homemade broth, such as Classic Chicken Bone Broth (page 113) and Long Run Mineral Broth (page 111), is superior in flavor and nutrition from boxed. If you're suffering from a common running ailment like inflammatory injuries, stress fractures, or digestive distress, making broth from scratch just might be your lifeline. Broth is an incredible, mineral-rich tonic that decreases inflammation, supports healthy bones, and aids recovery. Broth made from bones is rich in gelatin, which helps cure a range of digestive issues by coating the lining of the intestines, and is rich in glucosamine, chondroitin, calcium, and phosphorous—all essential nutrients for bone and joint health.

COCONUT

We have a slight obsession with coconut in all its glorious forms, including coconut water, coconut oil, coconut milk, dried coconut, and coconut sugar. We put coconut water (for an electrolyte boost) and coconut oil (for absorption of fat-soluble vitamins) in our smoothies, bake with coconut oil for its buttery richness, add shredded coconut to our granola to pack in the power, and stir coconut milk into everything from soups to curries.

Our love affair with coconut began long before we discovered its behind-the-scenes superpowers. But its powers are unbeatable: The medium chain fatty acid in coconut is a highly usable energy source, and it enhances our ability to absorb nutrients, stimulates metabolism, and boosts immunity.

When buying coconut oil, look for a brand labeled "virgin" and reach for organic coconut milk to avoid additives. Don't be tempted to buy the "light" stuff—it's just a watered-down version with the same price tag. When buying dried coconut flakes, check the label to make sure they're unsweetened.

DRIED FRUIT

We always have on hand an assortment of dried fruit—including dates, apricots, figs, and raisins—to toss into muffins or grain salads for a sweet burst or to snack on straight up with a handful of roasted nuts.

Dates make the ideal snack to fuel a long run since they're

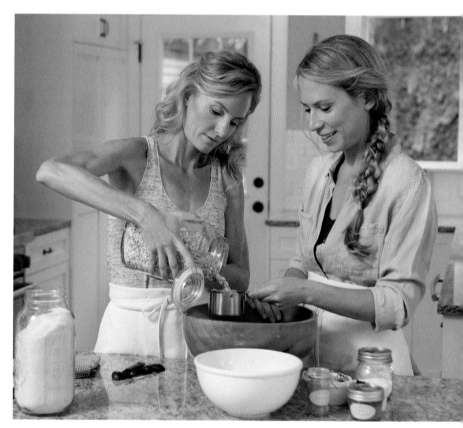

easy to digest and high in glucose for quick energy. And, unlike the processed glucose found in energy gels, they're naturally high in minerals, including potassium. Dates are the hero in our Giddy-Up Energy Bites (page 57).

Raisins are another favorite since they're rich in iron and B vitamins, essential nutrients for athletes. And dried figs satisfy a sweet craving, while aiding digestion with a beneficial dose of fiber. When buying dried fruit, check the label. The only ingredient should be the fruit.

FLOURS

Our favorite flours for baking wholesome treats are teff, dark rye, oat, spelt, and almond flour. Whole grain flours like teff and rye, unlike commercial wheat flour, aren't stripped of the germ and bran prior to grinding, making them an incredible source of nutrients. Teff flour is a nutritional powerhouse. It's packed with fiber, protein, iron, calcium, and more.

Almond flour is our go-to for the rich, buttery texture it gives to baked treats. We can feel good about devouring our baked goods made with almond flour since they're high in healthy fats, calcium, magnesium, and potassium. If you have a high-speed blender or food processor, you can easily grind your own almond flour for superior flavor and nutrition.

GRAINS

Whole grains are our jam. Look inside our pantries and you'll find jars of farro, quinoa, millet, short-grain brown rice, wild rice, steel-cut oats, and rolled oats. Although quinoa is technically not a grain (it's a seed), we've grouped it here since it cooks like a grain.

Whole grains are essential for vegetarians and vegans since they're rich in B vitamins and form a complete protein when eaten in combination with beans. Whole grains are a fantastic sustainable energy source for athletes since they're high in complex carbohydrates and are slow to digest.

Toss cooked farro, wild rice, or quinoa into a salad to transform it into a meal. Top brown or wild rice with cooked veggies and a sauce for a quick weeknight dinner. Bake with whole grain flours (see more on this in "Flours" on this page).

Cook grains in large batches and freeze individual portions after 4 or 5 days. Grains can be hard to digest for those not used to high fiber. Soaking them prior to cooking helps; so does cooking them with a piece of kombu (see "Sea Vegetables" on page 16).

LEGUMES (BEANS)

When beans are consumed in combination with a whole grain like rice, they form a complete protein, making them an essential food for vegetarian runners. Even nonvegetarians should consider including beans in their diet since they're high in B vitamins, folate, magnesium, zinc, and iron—all essential nutrients for energy. Beans are also proven to be protective against antioxidant damage. Bonus!

We keep a colorful assortment of dried beans stocked in glass jars, including chickpeas (garbanzo), green and red lentils, black beans, adzuki, and cannellini beans. We also keep canned beans on hand for quick weeknight meals.

Dried beans that are cooked properly are easier to digest than canned. We recommend soaking them overnight, then draining them. Place them in a pot, cover with fresh water, and simmer with a piece of kombu (see "Sea Vegetables" on page 16) until soft.

NUTS AND SEEDS

We're almost embarrassed by how many nuts we go through on a weekly basis. Almonds, walnuts, hazelnuts, cashews, and peanuts are all our friends. We grind them into flour for baking, roast them for salads, puree them for sauces, turn them into nut butter or nut milk, or simply roast them with a little olive oil and sea salt for instant snacking satisfaction.

Lucky for us nuts are a great source of heart-healthy fats, muscle-loving amino acids, and bone-building minerals, making them an ideal recovery snack. And we won't forget our equal love of seeds, especially sesame seeds and pumpkin seeds, which are rich in iron, zinc, calcium, magnesium, and potassium.

To save on cost, we like to buy nuts and seeds in bulk and store them in airtight glass jars in the pantry. Since the oils in nuts can go rancid, we recommend storing any amounts that you won't be consuming within a couple of months in the freezer.

OLIVE OIL

A high-quality olive oil is worth its weight in gold for its ability to transform the simplest dish and for its health-giving properties. Olive oil is a heart-healthy, monounsaturated fat, and its anti-inflammatory powers make it an ideal fat for runners to include in their diets every day. Studies show that 2 tablespoons of olive oil combats inflammation better than a dose of ibuprofen—and it definitely tastes better.

Stick to extra-virgin olive oil, which means the oil came from the first cold-pressing of the olives. We keep on hand two versions—a lighter, less expensive bottle for cooking and a bolder, more expensive bottle for homemade salad dressings, hummus, pesto, and baguette dunking. Olive oil should never be used in high-heat cooking. For stir-frying, we prefer to use a small amount of safflower oil since it has a high smoke point.

PASTA

What runner doesn't love pasta?! And we say if you're gonna eat pasta, eat real pasta. We keep boxes of durum wheat or semolina flour pasta on hand for the best flavor and texture.

Pasta perfection starts with correctly cooking the noodles. Pasta should be cooked in a large pot of heavily salted water that is brought to a full boil prior to adding the noodles. Check for doneness a couple of minutes prior to the cook time listed on the package to achieve that perfect al dente texture. You want your spaghetti to have some chew, not go all limp when drowned in sauce.

Speaking of sauce, we take our sauce-to-pasta ratio to the extreme. Since most of the good stuff is in the sauce—meat, veggies, and seasonings—we

prefer less pasta but lots of hearty sauce.

SARDINES (CANNED)

Keep a few cans of these oily little fish around for an instant power meal. Years ago we swapped our tuna habit for sardines for good reasons. They're lower in toxins and better for the environment and have a superior nutrition profile.

Sardines are one of the richest sources of B_{12} and B_6 (essential nutrients for fighting fatigue), inflammation-fighting omega-3s, calcium, and mood-boosting vitamin D. Because they're low on the food chain, they're also one of the cleanest fish you can get. Elyse brings along a can of sardines on picnics and camping trips since they're an absolute favorite food of her toddler.

SEA SALT

Sea salt deserves its own heading. Seriously it's your new best friend. Salt is essential for bringing out the flavor in food and shouldn't be feared in the kitchen. If you're avoiding processed foods, you don't need to worry about having too much sodium in your diet (unless you have a health condition). For runners, salt is essential for electrolyte balance.

Not all salts are created equal. Top-quality salts taste better because they're richer in essential trace minerals. Look for gray-hued Celtic sea salt or pink-hued Himalayan salt. For accuracy in measurements, we mostly use fine sea salt in this book, but a coarse sea salt is fabulous for a finishing touch.

SEA VEGETABLES (SEAWEED)

Seaweed is one of the most nutritionally dense foods on the planet (no wonder the Japanese have one of the highest life expectancies). Sea vegetables have more iron than red meat and 10 times the calcium of cow's milk. They're rich in B_{12}, making them a great food for vegans, and are high in electrolytes, a bonus for endurance athletes.

Our favorite dried sea vegetables—wakame, kombu, and nori—can be found in the ethnic food aisle at most natural foods stores or at any Asian market. Adding a small piece of kombu to a pot of simmering grains or beans imparts minerals and aids with digestion (discard the kombu after simmering). When it comes to consuming seaweed, a little goes a long way.

SEASONINGS

Bring on the spices, dried herbs, and vinegars! Learning how to play with seasonings makes everything in the kitchen more fun. Not only do seasonings add tons of flavor, they're also potent anti-inflammatories and digestion enhancers and are rich in minerals such as iron, magnesium, and calcium. Who knew?

We recommend buying spices and herbs in small quantities from the bulk bins at a store with high turnover. It's less expensive, and spices definitely lose their potency the longer they sit on the shelf. For storage, get a set of little glass jars that you can reuse.

Our loyal seasonings that you'll find most often in this book are oregano, fennel seeds, cumin, turmeric, red pepper flakes, cayenne, chile powder, bay leaves, and whole black peppercorns (definitely grind your pepper fresh). The sweet spices we adore are cinnamon, nutmeg, cloves, cardamom, and ginger.

We also keep on hand real soy sauce (shoyu or tamari is the way to go), pickled peppers, vinegars, and spicy Dijon mustard. Our top vinegar picks are balsamic vinegar and apple cider vinegar. When buying balsamic, check the label: It should say 100% balsamic vinegar. Many balsamic vinegars are just

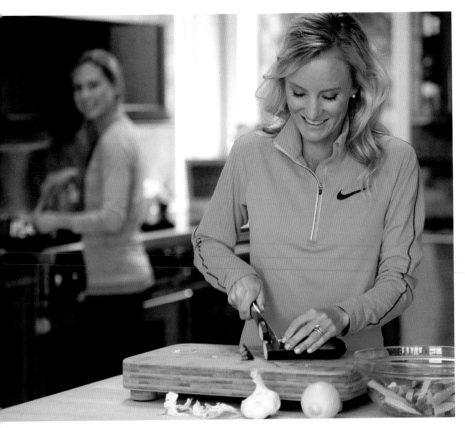

wine vinegar with caramel coloring and other additives. A true balsamic vinegar is expensive but a little goes a long way. For apple cider vinegar, seek out an unfiltered, organic brand that's cloudy and murky—that's the good stuff from natural fermentation. Apple cider vinegar is rich in probiotics and enzymes and great for digestion, which is a bonus for runners wanting to maximize nutrient absorption.

SWEETENERS

Sweet tooth? No problem. You can avoid refined cane sugar and still satisfy a sweet craving with any of our wholesome treat recipes, which are sweetened with honey, maple syrup, molasses, or coconut sugar. These are our preferred sweeteners because they're less processed,

mineral rich, and lower on the glycemic load. They also provide sustainable energy, and a little goes a long way. When buying honey, the darker the color the better. For maple syrup, we prefer grade B (dark amber) from Canada or Vermont. For molasses, go for black strap—the sticky, rich good stuff that's left over after the sugar crystals are extracted from cane sugar, making it crazy-high in iron.

Even though these sweeteners are less refined than white sugar, we still keep our consumption in check. We love our baked goods because they're balanced with whole grains and healthy fats and are considerably less sweet than store-bought baked goods. If you're used to eating more sugary treats, it might take some time

for your taste buds to adjust to our sweet style.

TOMATOES (CANNED OR CARTON)

Canned tomatoes (whole, crushed, or diced) are a must for making a quick marinara sauce or for adding depth to soups, stews, and chili. In the summer, we use fresh local tomatoes, but come winter, canned tomatoes are light-years better than anything you'll find in the produce section. Look for organic tomatoes in BPA-free cans or cartons.

Like everything else, the quality of canned tomatoes varies tremendously. If you're using a less expensive brand to make sauce, the tomatoes will taste more acidic, and you'll likely have to add a little sweetener at the end.

FRIDGE STAPLES

BUTTER

It's your lucky day because we're about to convince you that butter is a superfood. It's one of our favorite healthy fats because it's high in fat-soluble vitamins, including vitamins A, E, and K. Vitamin K doesn't get much publicity, but it's an essential nutrient for helping the body absorb calcium (stress fractures begone!).

When we say butter, we're talking real butter, from pastured cows, not margarine and definitely not vegan butter-flavored spreads. Butter tastes rich because it is rich—rich in fat-soluble vitamins and viable energy. Butter from grass-fed cows is a fantastic source of conjugated linoleic acid (CLA), a powerhouse fatty acid proven to help muscles recover faster. But

don't reach for the supplemental form of CLA, which is highly processed and often derived from cheap vegetable oils.

There's a reason why cooking with fat makes everything taste better. Fat is a carrier for flavor and also a carrier for all the fat-soluble vitamins that your hard-working body craves. So now you know why a smear of butter is so incredibly satisfying.

For the freshest taste, store unused sticks of butter in your freezer and store only what you need for the week in the fridge. We use unsalted butter when baking to give accurate salt measurements in the recipes, but if your butter is salted, just cut down on the amount of salt given in the recipe. If you're sensitive to dairy, try cultured butter, which has less lactose.

CARROTS

Carrots provide an essential sweet component and aromatics when combined with onions in a wide range of recipes. We also love tossing carrots into smoothies and grating them into salads or even muffins.

Heart-healthy carrots are rich in antioxidant nutrients, including beta-carotene (vitamin A), vitamin K, vitamin C, and minerals, especially potassium.

Peel your carrots to avoid the bitter flavor in the skin. Carrots stay fresh for several weeks when stored in a sealed bag in a drawer in the fridge. If you buy your carrots with the tops intact, remove the greens prior to storage.

CHEESE (PARMESAN, GOAT CHEESE, FETA)

Since living abroad in Switzerland, Elyse is particular about her cheeses. Not all cheeses are created equal. You won't find blocks of orange cheddar cheese in our fridge, but you will find a regular rotation of aged Parmesan, creamy goat cheese (chèvre), sheep's milk feta, and raw milk aged Gruyère.

Parmesan is a must. It adds a salty richness to dishes and can transform nearly anything. We love it on salads, soups, and pasta. It's high in calcium and vitamin K_2, two essentials for cardiovascular and bone health. Seriously, do not buy that powdery stuff that comes in a canister (or if you do, don't tell us!). Buy aged Parmesan in a wedge right off the wheel and grate it fresh. If wrapped tightly in plastic and stored in the fridge, it keeps for months (but we haven't tested this because it never lasts longer than a week in our homes).

If you're sensitive to dairy like so many runners are, you'll be thrilled to discover that goat cheese and aged cheeses are a lot easier to digest than processed American cheese.

EGGS

If you've got a carton of eggs in your fridge, you're set to whip together an easy and incredibly nourishing breakfast, lunch, or dinner. We eat eggs fried, scrambled, soft-boiled, or hard-boiled and use them in quiches, frittatas, omelets, rice dishes, baked goods, and more.

Eggs have all nine amino acids, making them an easily assimi-lated, complete protein and a source of B_{12} and vitamin D. Don't toss the yolk since the majority of the nutrients and heart-healthy fat are in the yellow. We prefer to buy our eggs at the farmers' market since truly pastured eggs are richer in vitamins (and flavor). Pastured means the chicken is free to roam and forage bugs and grasses all day. Many of the labels on eggs at the supermarket, like "cage-free" and "free-range," don't tell the full story. An egg can be labeled "free-range" if the chicken is simply given a tiny plot of barren land next to its cage.

GARLIC

Garlic has been used for centuries not only to add zest to an array of dishes but also for medicinal purposes. Garlic is a potent antibacterial and is proven to boost virus-fighting T-cells, making it a best friend of our immune system. Studies also show that garlic may help boost iron absorption and cardiovascular health, both critical functions for runners.

Raw garlic is the way to go to cash in on its health-giving properties (that is, as long as you're not heading out on a date!). Store garlic bulbs in a dark, ventilated place, not your fridge.

It's a rare day that we aren't using garlic in some form. We put it in salad dressings, pesto, hummus, guacamole, sauces, soups, stews, stir-fries, pasta—the list goes on.

GINGER

We have a slight obsession with ginger. Its versatility and incredible sweet-spiciness is why you'll find fresh ginger in a lot of our recipes. Not to mention that ginger is fabulous for digestion. It soothes the intestinal tract and helps eliminate gas. It's also a potent anti-inflammatory and an antioxidant powerhouse.

Fresh ginger is a must-have for smoothies, tea, soups, and even baked goods. You can find it in the produce section at most grocery stores. The root should be peeled (use the edge of a spoon) and grated (a microplane grater works well for this).

LEMONS

A bag of lemons should be in your fridge at all times. Adding a squeeze of lemon juice to many dishes will brighten the flavor and add depth. We love using fresh lemon juice in salad dressings and sauces, and the zest transforms baked goods.

Start your day with a hydrating, alkalizing, vitamin-C-rich, digestion-stimulating tonic by sipping warm water with fresh lemon juice.

MISO

A dollop of miso paste adds a rich, salty, umami flavor to dressings, soups, and savory dishes. For those avoiding dairy, it's a great substitute for Parmesan cheese since it has a similar flavor profile. Miso is incredible for runners because it's rich in probiotics and enzymes to help build good gut flora for better digestion.

Miso is traditionally made from fermented soybeans, but you can find soy-free versions such as chickpea miso. Our favorite varieties are white miso for its versatility and mild flavor and barley miso for soup. You can find miso paste at any natural foods store or Asian market—even at some grocery stores. Our favorite brand for its rich flavor and traditional aging process is Miso Master, which you can find at www.great-eastern-sun.com.

ONIONS

Onions are the jumping-off point for the majority of savory dishes and simply cannot be overlooked. The varieties of onions we always have on hand are yellow onions and shallots. We also love red onions and green onions (scallions) for spiking salads and soups.

The onion's potent, mouth-watering flavor comes from its sulfur-containing compounds and its flavonoids. Onions are rich in B vitamins and antioxidants. They are in the same family as garlic and similarly are known for their ability to boost immunity and fight inflammation.

Onions with edible green tops—like green onions, chives, and leeks—should be kept in the fridge, but onions with papery skins should be stored in a dark, ventilated place (think basement).

TEMPEH

If you're looking for a healthy alternative to meat, give tempeh a try. Tempeh is made by fermenting whole, cooked soybeans and is healthier than tofu since it's far less processed. The fermentation process makes tempeh easier to digest and the nutrients more bioavailable—a good thing since it's rich in calcium, manganese, magnesium, copper, iron, and vitamin B_2.

Tempeh doesn't taste like much right out of the package, but it will happily soak up the flavor of any marinade or sauce that you cook it in. Tempeh should be stored in the fridge and can be frozen if not used by the sell-by-date.

WHOLE MILK YOGURT

Plain, whole milk, organic yogurt is your best bet when buying yogurt. It's lower in sugar and higher in satisfying, energizing fat, not to mention way better tasting and less processed than low-fat flavored yogurts.

We often substitute yogurt for mayonnaise in recipes such

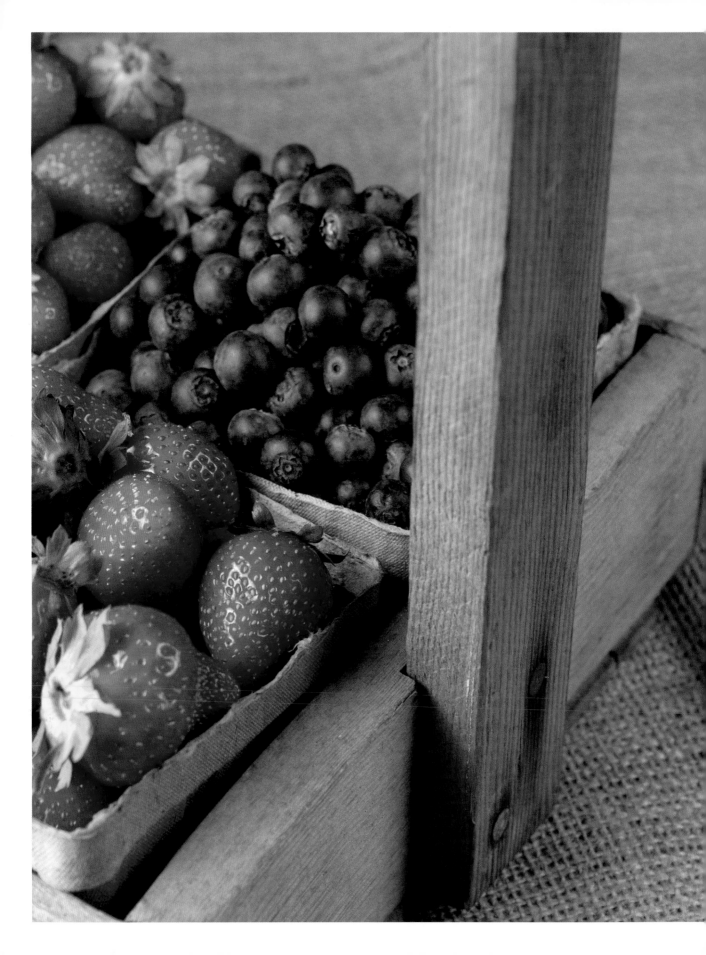

as egg and chicken salad, and we love to use it in place of cream in baked goods. Yogurt, since it's fermented, is easier to digest than cream and is a fabulous source of probiotics for maintaining healthy gut flora. Yogurt is also rich in calcium, zinc, and vitamin B_{12}.

FRESH FAVORITES

Our diet varies greatly week to week, depending on what's in season, but here are a few of the favorites that make a regular appearance in our baskets.

APPLES AND PEARS

Rambling through the apple and pear orchards in Hood River is our favorite fall pastime. Come September you'll always find a basket of apples and pears on our counters. Shalane's go-to PM snack is an apple smeared with nut butter. We also keep apples on hand for tossing in smoothies, salads, yogurt muesli bowls, and desserts.

Apples and pears are rich in antioxidants, vitamin C, and fiber. Apples often get overlooked for fancier-sounding superfruits, but the ol' apple should not be forgotten.

ASPARAGUS

Asparagus are a happy bunch any way you want to cook them. Simply grill them or roast them with a little olive oil, salt, and pepper, and they'll shine. Or toss them into stir-fries, scrambled eggs, pastas, or salads.

Asparagus are at their prime in the springtime. They have a wealth of flavor and nutrients, with fiber for digestion, vitamin K for strong bones, B vitamins for energy, and vitamins A, C, and E.

AVOCADOS

Oh, how we adore this creamy fruit (yes, avocado is a fruit!). If we were stranded on an island with only an avocado tree, we would be able to survive. You can't beat half an avocado sprinkled with sea salt as an afternoon snack.

Avocados are rich in one of the healthiest fats out there: monounsaturated fatty acids, which are glorious for fighting inflammation. You'll find avocados snuck into recipes throughout this book for good reason. Their rich fat content makes it easier for the body to absorb fat-soluble nutrients, which is reason enough to add them to any veggie-loaded meal.

BANANAS

Bananas are a coveted food among runners the world over. Head to the food table at any race and you're bound to find a basket of halved bananas. Bananas naturally contain several essential nutrients for endurance athletes, including complex carbohydrates for fuel, potassium and other electrolytes for fluid balance and muscle contraction, and vitamin B_6 for energy metabolism.

Store bananas on your counter. If they get too ripe, peel them and freeze them for smoothies—or better yet, let them get really brown until you have no choice but to make banana bread.

BEEF, BISON

Peer into our freezers and you'll find a stash of ground beef and ground bison (aka buffalo). Grass-fed red meat is incredibly nourishing and satisfying. When Shalane is training at high-altitude, she finds herself craving burgers. That's because beef and bison are rich in iron, a mineral your red blood cells need to carry oxygen to your hardworking muscles. They're also rich in protein, omega-3 fatty acids, B vitamins, and CLA. (See "Butter" on page 17 to learn more about CLA.)

You don't need to eat beef every day to reap its benefits. We typically work it into our diets once or twice a week. Always seek out the highest quality possible. Meat from healthy, happy animals tastes better and is better for your body and the planet.

BEETS

Beet smoothies, beet hummus, pickled beets, roasted beets—we're red tuber-crazy around here. This sweet, earthy root is rich in antioxidants, anti-inflammatory compounds, and nitrites. Not the kind of nitrites in hot dogs, but naturally occurring nitric oxide, which is proven to lower blood pressure and may increase endurance.

Don't toss those beet greens. They're rich in calcium and have a mild flavor. Blend them into a smoothie or sauté them in a little olive oil with garlic, sea salt, and red pepper flakes. Separate the beet roots from the greens and store them in a plastic bag in the fridge. They'll stay fresh for 3 weeks, but the greens should be used within a few days.

BERRIES

From June through September, we live in berry bliss here in Oregon where a variety of berries grow on farms, in backyards, and along our favorite running trails. We try to pick and stockpile enough berries for the winter, but our stash never lasts long enough.

Blueberries, strawberries, and raspberries (Shalane's personal fave) pack a sweet punch of nutrients including antioxidants, anti-inflammatory compounds, vitamin C, folate, and potassium. Who needs a multivitamin when you've got a handful of fresh berries?

Berries are on the Dirty Dozen list for pesticide residue, so seek out organic or local berries from a trusted farm. Store them unwashed in a sealed bag in the fridge, or wash and dry them and freeze for smoothies and baked treats.

BREAD

Bread can be a healthy part of a whole foods diet if you know how to shop for the real deal. We almost always have a slice of bread from a crusty whole grain loaf with lunch or dinner. When buying bread, it's important to check the ingredients—or better yet, buy a fresh, artisan loaf from a local bakery.

Many store-bought breads are full of sugar, added gluten, nutrient-stripped flours, and preservatives. The additives are what keep a loaf of sandwich bread soft and fresh tasting for an entire week. Fresh-baked bread, on the other hand, only lasts for a couple of days, but don't let that deter you. You can slice off what you aren't going to use, wrap it in foil, put it in a plastic zip-top bag, and freeze

it. When shopping for a whole grain bread, keep in mind the ingredient list needs to actually say "whole wheat flour" not "wheat flour," which is equivalent to nutrient-stripped white flour.

BUTTERNUT SQUASH

Butternut squash is our favorite fall squash because of its versatility. Roast it and toss it into pasta, or add a little broth and puree it into a soup. There's a reason to load up on butternut when the weather changes. It's got the right mix of antioxidants and vitamin C to put up your best defense against cold and flu season.

Lucky for us, Elyse has a giant butternut squash vine growing in her front yard. Butternut squash stores extremely well and will stay fresh stored in a cool, dark place for months.

CAULIFLOWER

We used to think cauliflower was such a drab veggie, until we discovered its incredible transformation when roasted. Now we roast a batch nearly every week for a fabulous soup and salad topper. We also discovered that pulsing raw cauliflower florets in the food processor transforms it into the texture of couscous—a fabulous way to sneak more veggies into your family's dinner.

Cauliflower is a nutrient-dense cruciferous star. Studies show that the form of calcium in this veggie is easier to absorb than the calcium in milk.

CHICKEN (DARK MEAT)

Everyone knows chicken is a great source of protein. But did you know it's rich in minerals, especially iron, and vitamins such as energy-giving B vitamins?

When buying chicken, look for a pasture-raised or organic bird for superior flavor and nutrition. And don't pass over the dark meat—it's higher in fat (good fat!) and more mineral-dense than the breast. It's also less expensive and tastes better (remember fat is a carrier for flavor!).

CITRUS (ORANGES, GRAPEFRUIT)

In the winter, our philosophy is, "An orange (or grapefruit) a day keeps the doc away." Citrus fruits aren't just vitamin C powerhouses; the humble orange has more than 170 phytonutrients. These nutrients are fabulous for fighting inflammation, detoxing the body, maintaining a healthy pH level, boosting immunity, and enhancing cardiovascular health.

When peeling a grapefruit or orange, try to leave as much of the pith as possible. A lot of the fruit's nutrients hang out in this

inner skin. In college we drank gallons of store-bought OJ until we found out how processed it is. Even the cartons labeled 100% OJ pale in comparison to fresh-squeezed juice. Now our go-to juicy remedy is what we call Whole Fruit Juice (see recipes on page 33).

If you're looking for a healthier alternative to your sports drink, try a combination of fresh-squeezed OJ, coconut water, filtered water, and a pinch of sea salt—energizing hydration that tastes phenomenal!

FISH

Fish makes at least a weekly appearance in our diets. It's an easily digestible source of protein and is also rich in inflammation-fighting omega-3 fatty acids, energizing B vitamins, bone-building magnesium, and other essential minerals.

Our household favorites here in Oregon are wild salmon, halibut, and Pacific cod. Since salmon is often overfished, a fantastic alternative is arctic char.

Our meat philosophy applies to seafood as well: We would rather eat the best quality, sustainable seafood, pay more for it, and eat less of it than fill up on toxin-loaded, factory-farmed fish. We highly recommend consulting SeafoodWatch.org to find the best options in your area.

GREENS (SPINACH, KALE, BROCCOLI, ARUGULA)

Popeye was on to something when he attributed his strength to eating spinach. If only we had more veggie-loving cartoon characters to influence our kids to eat their greens. Greens of all shapes and sizes—including spinach, kale, broccoli, arugula, collards, and Brussels sprouts—are packed with more nutrients than we have room to list here.

If you're looking to get more greens into your diet, you've picked up the right cookbook. We love sneaking veggies into everything, from muffins and smoothies to soup, quiche, and even meatballs. Our lives would not be complete without them.

HERBS (BASIL, PARSLEY, CILANTRO)

Most home cooks skip the step of garnishing a dish with fresh herbs, but herbs like basil, parsley, and cilantro do a whole lot more than make a dish look pretty. They add freshness, another layer of enticing flavor, satisfying color, and an incredible set of phytonutrients.

Herbs are revered the world over for their antioxidant and anti-inflammatory benefits. If you're running, jumping, swimming, or playing, your body is constantly breaking down and repairing cells. Herbs are a healing salve for those cells.

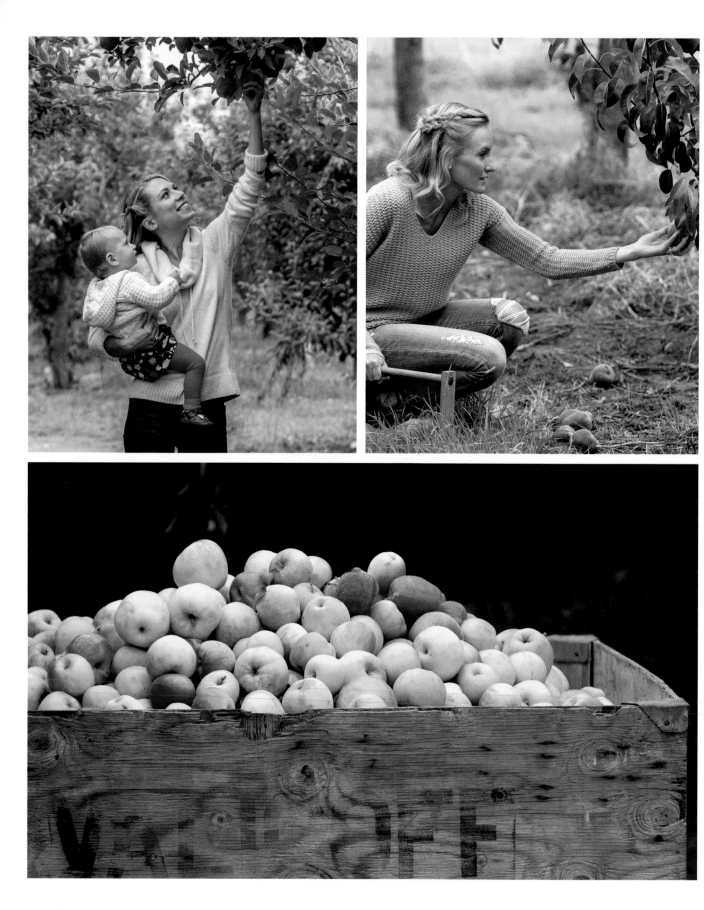

RUN FAST EAT SLOW

Use delicate herbs like basil, parsley, and cilantro to enhance salads and heartier herbs like oregano, thyme, and sage to add depth to cooked dishes. Keep herbs on hand by growing them at home. All you need is a few pots placed strategically in a sunny windowsill or a small plot in the backyard.

MUSHROOMS

The mysterious mushroom should not be passed by when making your rounds in the produce aisle. They add a satisfying meaty flavor and texture to vegetarian dishes and a satiating earthy sweetness. Our go-to varieties are cremini and shiitake.

If you aren't eating meat, you should consider adding mushrooms to your diet since they're a B and D vitamin powerhouse and are proven to boost immunity. There's a reason why the Chinese have used them in medicine for thousands of years. Mushrooms should be cooked, not eaten raw. They store best in a brown paper bag in the fridge.

STONE FRUIT (PEACHES, PLUMS, APRICOTS)

These coveted summer fruits are a sweet source of vitamins and minerals. They're rich in niacin, vitamin K, vitamin C, potassium, magnesium, and calcium. Peaches, plums, and apricots are fabulous eaten fresh and also shine in baked goods. When your favorite stone fruit is at its prime, slice it up and freeze it for smoothies, oatmeal, and future pies.

Nothing beats sinking your teeth into a ripe peach after a long run on a hot summer day, except maybe slurping a big bite of cool watermelon. (Side note: Shalane doesn't like watermelon—shocking!—which is why you won't find watermelon in this book. Just sneaking in a mention here: Watermelon is a glorious food for runners).

SWEET POTATOES (YAMS)

We are madly in love with this vibrant, nourishing, orange root. Lucky for us sweet potatoes taste delicious year-round and are a dependable, versatile option for a fast, healthy dinner. We hope you like sweet potatoes as much as we do because this tuber has infiltrated many recipes in our book. (Sweet Potato Breakfast Cookies? Yes, please! See page 56.)

The variety of sweet potatoes best for baking and roasting is the orange-fleshed sweet potatoes often labeled "yams" at grocery stores. Yams are our top pick for a prerace dinner since they're an easily digestible source of complex carbs and protein. Make your marathon carbo-loading count!

TOMATOES

We covet tomatoes in the summer months when they're sweet, juicy, and vibrant and require little effort to transform into a meal. We like them best sliced thin and topped with olive oil, balsamic vinegar, fresh basil, mozzarella, and sea salt.

Tomatoes are rich in cancer-fighting and cardio-boosting lycopene, and they deliver a wealth of B vitamins that are associated with energy and focus. Everything you need to keep your eye on the competition.

Once you eat a backyard or farmers' market tomato, you'll never be able to go back to the flavorless, mealy ones on most grocery stores shelves. Tomatoes lose flavor and texture in the fridge. They should be left out on the counter and eaten within a couple of days.

Ready to roll? Let's get cooking!

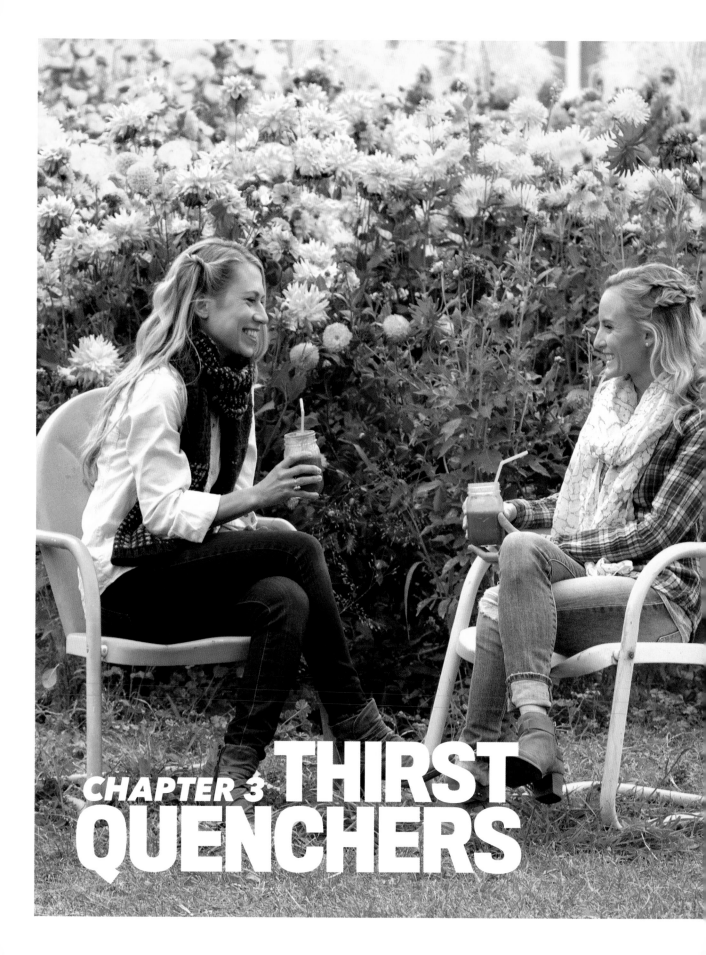

CHAPTER 3 THIRST QUENCHERS

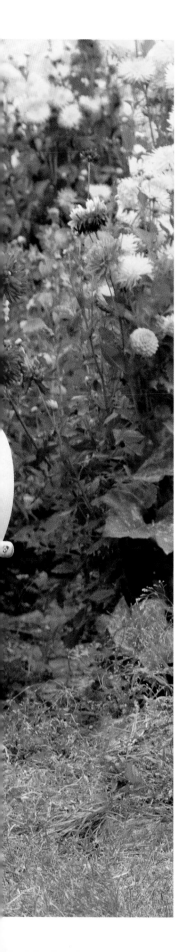

CAN'T BEET ME SMOOTHIE

SERVES 2

for speed-workout days

If you have a high-speed blender such as a Vitamix, you don't need to cook the beet. Using it raw preserves nutrients, and it will puree completely in the blender. Simply peel and quarter.

Don't put those beet greens in the compost pile! They're chock-full of inflammation-fighting nutrients. Use them in stir-fries, pasta, or pesto (page 67) or toss them right into the smoothie.

Beets continue to gain respect among runners for their performance-enhancing benefits—and for good reason. Beets are packed with nutrients and are rich in antioxidants and minerals, all good things for your cardiovascular health.

Since Elyse couldn't convince Shalane to eat a big beet salad for breakfast, this beet-rich smoothie is how Shalane now fuels up before a hard morning workout. The coconut water gives a boost of electrolytes, and the almond butter helps her body absorb the fat-soluble vitamins in the beets and blueberries.

Shalane shared this recipe with elite marathoner Matt Llano while they were training together in Flagstaff, and this has become his go-to smoothie.

This recipe makes enough for two, so your running buddy can fuel up, too. Or you can store leftovers in the fridge for up to 3 days.

---

1 cooked beet (see directions opposite), peeled and quartered

1 cup frozen blueberries

1 small frozen banana

1 cup unsweetened almond milk or other milk of choice (Homemade Hazelnut Milk, page 34)

1 cup coconut water

1-inch knob fresh ginger, peeled (use edge of a spoon)

1 tablespoon almond butter

1. In a blender, place the beet, blueberries, banana, milk, coconut water, ginger, and almond butter. Blend on high speed for several minutes until smooth.

2. For rushed mornings, this smoothie can be made the night before. Simply stir in the a.m. and sip while you lace up.

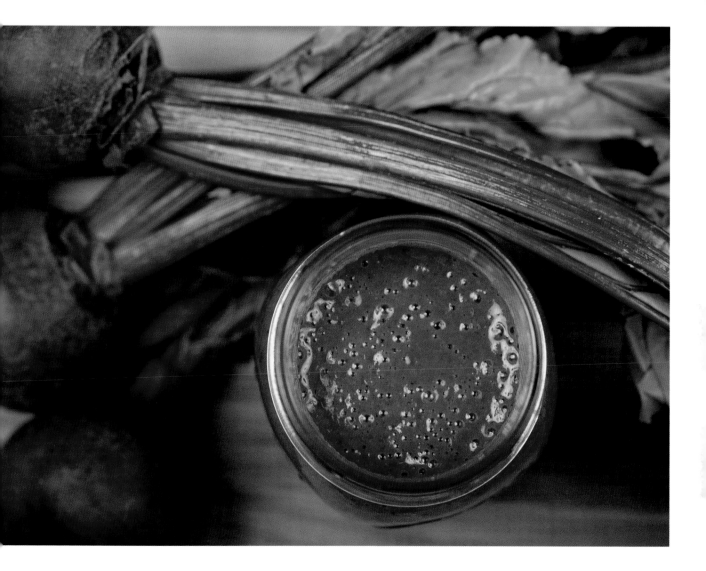

TWO EASY METHODS TO COOK BEETS

Oven

Wrap unpeeled, trimmed beets individually in foil and place
on a rimmed baking sheet. Roast in the oven at 350°F for
1 to 1½ hours, depending on the size. Beets are done when a
butter knife easily pierces through the center of each beet.
Cool, peel, and store in the fridge for up to 5 days.

Stovetop

Place trimmed beets in a small pot, cover with water, and bring
to a boil over high heat. Reduce the heat to low and simmer until a
butter knife easily pierces through the center of each beet, 25 to
35 minutes. Cool, peel, and store in the fridge for up to 5 days.

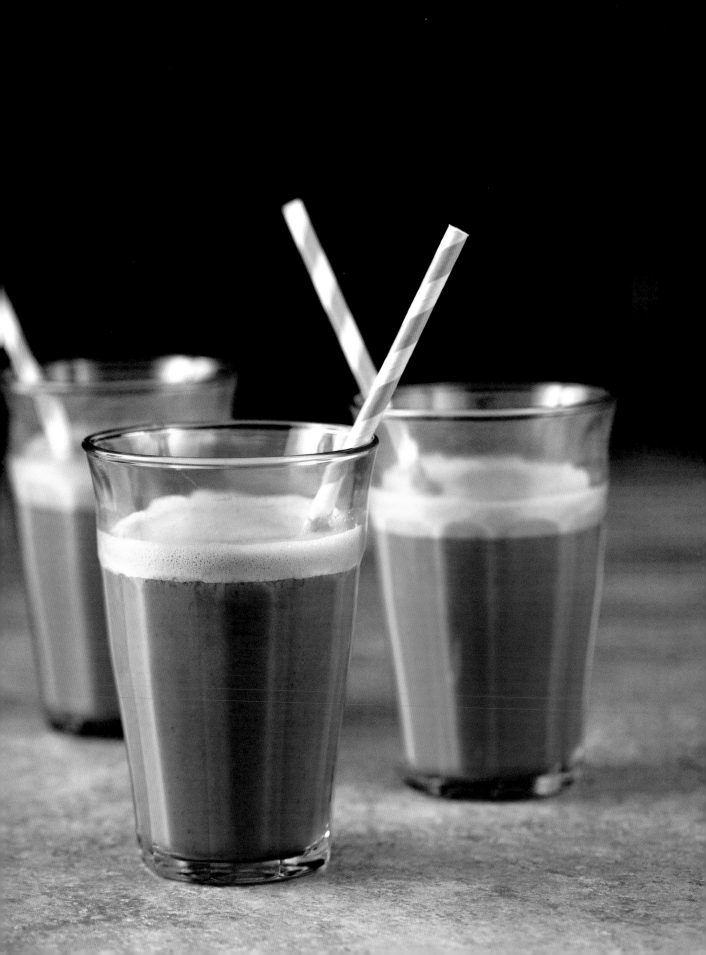

COCONUT-KALE SMOOTHIE

SERVES 2

for going the extra mile

Portland is a small city packed to the brim with creative people churning out incredible food. Lucky for us, you don't have to go to a fancy restaurant to experience an inspiring dish. In fact, some of our favorite spots to chow down at are the endless food carts. And one of our favorite carts to cruise by when we're in need of a health fix is the Kure Juice Bar.

This recipe is inspired by our go-to smoothie at the Kure. Not surprisingly, it's called the Extra Mile. One sip of this refreshing, mean-green smoothie and you'll be ready to go that extra mile.

A high-speed blender will achieve the creamiest results.

---

4 kale leaves, stems removed

2 cups coconut water

½ cup whole milk yogurt

2 tablespoons almond butter

3 or 4 dates, pitted, or
1 to 2 tablespoons honey

1 cup ice

In a blender, place the kale, coconut water, yogurt, almond butter, dates or honey, and ice. Blend on high speed for several minutes until smooth.

GREEN TEA-GREEN APPLE SMOOTHIE

SERVES 2

for an immediate energy boost

In the summer, make a big batch of iced green tea for energizing sipping. We like to add fresh mint into our brew.

This cool green smoothie is refreshing and energizing and packs a mean punch of antioxidants and vitamins from squeezing three green powerhouses into one glass: green tea, green apple, and kale. Adding a superb fat (peanut butter, in this case) will give you lasting power and helps your body better absorb the incredible fat-soluble nutrients.

For an afternoon pick-me-up on days when we need a little dose of caffeine but don't want to overdo it with the coffee, this is our rescue remedy.

For the juiciest results, a high-speed blender is preferred.

---

1 cup unsweetened green tea, cold or at room temperature

1 cup unsweetened almond milk or other milk of choice (Homemade Hazelnut Milk, page 34)

1 green apple, quartered and core removed

1 large kale leaf, stem removed, or beet greens (see page 22)

3 to 5 dates, depending on sweetness preference

2 tablespoons creamy peanut butter

¼ teaspoon ground cinnamon (optional)

1 cup ice

In a blender, place the green tea, milk, apple, kale or beet greens, dates, peanut butter, cinnamon (if using), and ice. Blend on high speed for several minutes until smooth.

WHOLE FRUIT JUICE

for a head start to the day

Hear us out. Bottled 100% orange juice sounds healthy, but it is highly processed and pasteurized, meaning less nutrition, zero fiber, zero enzymes, and a whole lotta sugar. Not the best way to start your day.

Years ago we gave up our habit of drinking OJ first thing in the morning and replaced it with this hydrating formula below. We call these juices Whole Fruit Juice because, unlike store-bought juice, all the incredible edible parts of the fruits and vegetables are used. This means you're giving your body more of the good stuff and wasting less. In fact, the healthiest part of grapefruits and oranges is the pith, which is full of beneficial fiber and vitamins.

Drink these juices before breakfast to get a head start on your fruit and veggie fix for the day. We highly recommend using a high-speed blender to achieve smooth results.

Grapefruit Carrot Berry
SERVES 2

1 grapefruit, outer peel and seeds removed

2 small carrots or 1 large, peeled and halved

½ cup frozen blueberries or strawberries

2 cups coconut water

1-inch knob ginger, peeled (optional)

In a high-speed blender, place the grapefruit, carrots, berries, coconut water, and ginger (if using). Blend on high speed for several minutes until smooth.

 Add a spoonful of virgin coconut oil to make it easier for your body to absorb the fat-soluble vitamins.

Orange Carrot Mango
SERVES 2

2 oranges, outer peel and seeds removed

2 small carrots or 1 large, peeled and halved

½ cup frozen mango or pineapple chunks

2 cups coconut water or filtered water

1-inch knob ginger, peeled (optional)

In a high-speed blender, place the oranges, carrots, mango or pineapple, coconut water, and ginger (if using). Blend on high speed for several minutes until smooth.

Don't have coconut water? Use filtered water and add a few pitted dates instead, to add the same refreshing sweetness.

HOMEMADE HAZELNUT MILK

MAKES ABOUT 5 CUPS

for a nondairy milk

Don't toss the protein- and fiber-rich leftover pulp. It can be stored in the freezer and tossed into smoothies, muffins, and more!

Since cow's milk and soy milk can be hard to digest, almond or hazelnut milk is our drink of choice for adding to coffee, tea, oatmeal, and smoothies (or savoring on its own!). The trouble with store-bought nut milk is it tastes like the cardboard package it comes in unless you buy the sugar-loaded vanilla variation. While studying at the Natural Gourmet Institute in New York City, Elyse got hooked on making almond milk. It's incredibly creamy, rich, and satisfying.

Upon returning to Oregon, Elyse started making her nut milk with hazelnuts (99 percent of the US crop of hazelnuts comes from our home state of Oregon!) and discovered an even more swoon-worthy beverage. (It's so good that Elyse's 6-year-old niece calls it a milkshake.) Our favorite late-night snack is a bowl of Ginger-Molasses Granola (page 54) drowned in this milk.

This recipe requires advance prep. For the creamiest results (and to maximize the digestibility), soak the nuts overnight.

1½ cups hazelnuts

4 cups cold filtered water

1 teaspoon vanilla extract or 1 whole vanilla bean, slit vertically to open

4 or 5 dates, pitted, or 2 to 3 tablespoons maple syrup

½ teaspoon ground cinnamon (optional)

¼ teaspoon fine sea salt

1. Place the hazelnuts in a large glass jar and fill with enough water to cover. Soak for at least 4 hours or overnight. Strain the nuts and rinse under fresh water.

2. Place the nuts and filtered water in a high-speed blender. Secure the lid and slowly increase the speed to the blender's highest setting and whir for 1 to 2 minutes until smooth and creamy.

3. Rinse a 12-inch piece of cheesecloth in cold water and wring it out. Fold in half and place as a liner in a mesh sieve. Over a bowl, pour a small amount of nut mixture through the sieve and squeeze the cheesecloth to extract as much liquid as possible. Set aside the pulp (see the Gold Medal tip above) and continue to pour small amounts through the cheesecloth-lined sieve until all the milk is extracted. (To make it easier, it's worth purchasing a nut milk bag.)

4. Give the blender a quick rinse and pour the hazelnut milk back into it. Add the vanilla extract or vanilla bean seeds, the dates or maple syrup, cinnamon (if using), and salt. Blend briefly until combined.

5. Pour the milk into a quart-size glass jar, seal, and store in the fridge for up to 3 days.

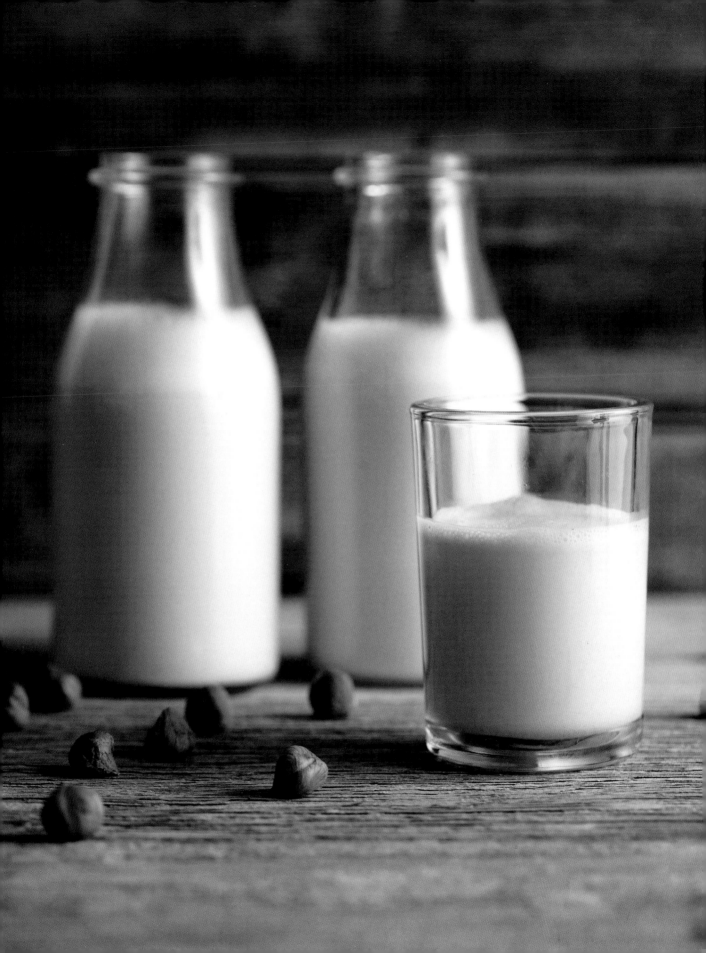

RUNNER'S RECOVERY ICED TEA

MAKES 25 CUPS OF TEA

for a mineral-rich brew

For this recipe, we consulted with Dr. JJ Pursell, author of *The Herbal Apothecary: 100 Medicinal Herbs and How to Use Them* and owner of Fettle Botanic Supply & Counsel in Portland, Oregon, and Brooklyn, New York. We sought out her expertise to help us craft a nourishing, mineral-rich tonic for athletes to sip after an all-out training session. We also asked her to hand-select her favorite dried herbs for battling common running ailments, including digestive distress, inflammation, and stress.

The end result is this refreshing hibiscus and lemongrass herbal tea with alfalfa, horsetail, and chamomile. Because it tastes citrusy, juicy, and naturally sweet, we know you'll remember to brew and sip often. Combine the herbs in a tea tin or small glass jar, and you've got your new favorite herbal tea blend at the ready for brewing a single cup any time of day.

To learn more about the benefits of each of these herbs, read the descriptions on the opposite page. These herbs can be found at herbal tea specialty shops or at fettlebotanic.com.

½ cup (1.125 ounces) dried hibiscus

¼ cup (.25 ounce) dried chamomile

2 tablespoons (.25 ounce) dried lemongrass

2 tablespoons (.125 ounce) dried alfalfa

1 tablespoon (.125 ounce) dried horsetail

Honey (optional)

1. Place the hibiscus, chamomile, lemongrass, alfalfa, and horsetail in a pint-size glass jar or tea tin, and shake until evenly combined.

2. Place 1 to 2 teaspoons of the herb blend in a tea infuser or tea ball, and steep in 8 ounces hot water for 8 to 10 minutes. Remove the tea infuser, stir in a little honey to taste (if using), and serve over ice.

3. For a medicinal-strength tea, place 4 tablespoons of the herb blend in a quart-size mason jar. Fill the jar with 4 cups hot but not boiling water. Cover and allow the herbs to steep for 1 hour or overnight. Strain using a fine mesh sieve and serve over ice.

4. Store the leftover herbal tea blend in an airtight container for up to 3 months.

NOTE: While this formula is generally regarded as very safe, we are all individuals and can react differently to herbs. Consult with your doctor prior to sipping if you have any medical concerns or if you are pregnant or nursing.

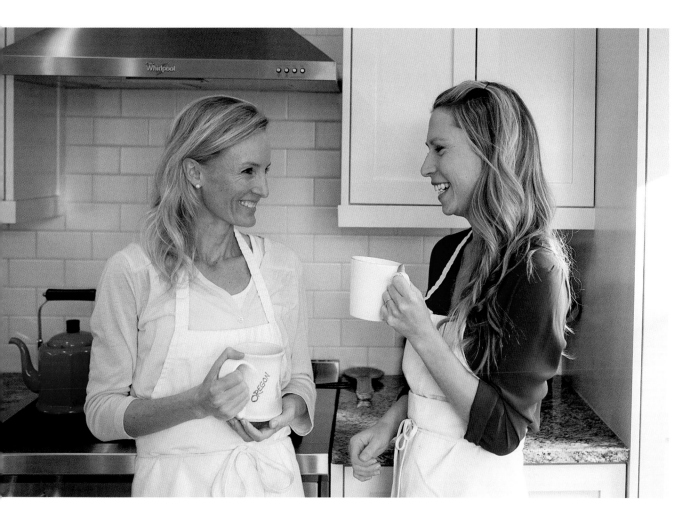

HIBISCUS
High in vitamin C and antioxidants, as well as iron, zinc, and phosphorus. Iron is crucial for the formation of red blood cells, which help your body absorb oxygen.

CHAMOMILE
Used in natural medicine for thousands of years to calm the nerves and soothe digestion.

LEMONGRASS
Super high in antioxidants and helps relax the nervous system by supporting the adrenal gland.

ALFALFA
Loaded with inflammation-fighting trace minerals.

HORSETAIL
Has inflammation-fighting trace minerals and helps the body store more calcium for bone strength.

ENERGIZING CHAI

MAKES 1 QUART

for lasting stamina

Energy drinks, step aside. This is what we sip to fuel our minds, bodies, and souls. Chai tea with all its warming spices is incredibly restorative and revitalizing. There's a reason why this beverage has been celebrated for more than 5,000 years and has a claim to fame as a healing drink in ancient Ayurvedic medicine.

Because we have a slight obsession with ginger in all its spicy, digestive-enhancing glory, we make our chai extra gingery. Feel free to scale up or down to your liking.

To give our chai an Oregonian twist, we like it best swirled with Homemade Hazelnut Milk (page 34). Learn more about Oregon's incredible hazelnuts on page 34, as well.

3 cups filtered water

2-inch knob fresh ginger, peeled and roughly grated

6 cardamom pods, crushed

3 whole cloves

1 cinnamon stick

3 black or green tea bags or 1 tablespoon loose-leaf black or green tea, placed in a tea ball

1½ cups Homemade Hazelnut Milk (page 34) or other milk of choice

Honey or coconut sugar

1. In a medium pot, combine the water, ginger, cardamom, cloves, and cinnamon. Bring to a boil, then reduce the heat to low, cover, and simmer for 15 minutes.

2. Turn off the heat, add the tea bags or tea ball, cover, and steep for 5 minutes.

3. Remove the tea, add the milk, sweeten to your liking with honey or coconut sugar, and heat just until warm. Pour through a strainer into 4 mugs.

4. For iced chai, skip warming the milk. Sweeten, strain, and pour over ice.

5. Store leftovers in a quart-size glass jar in the fridge.

APPLE-GINGER CIDER

SERVES 2

for postwinter run hydration

This drink is delicious served cold. Pour the cider into a glass jar and allow it to cool. Serve diluted to half strength with sparkling mineral water.

At the base of Mount Hood just outside of Portland, Oregon, there's an incredibly scenic valley of rolling farmland called Hood River. Aptly dubbed the "Fruit Loop," Hood River is one of the nation's largest apple-growing regions. Come fall, a favorite pastime for Portlanders is an excursion to the valley's farms to pick apples and bring home a gallon or two of fresh-pressed juice.

Also in fall the rain returns to Oregon. After being spoiled by a summer of sunny days, it can be hard to get out the door for a long run in a cold drizzle. To help with motivation, Elyse created this enticing mug of goodness to look forward to after sliding around in the mud. The sweet cinnamon and spicy ginger are remarkable anti-inflammatory and digestion-enhancing aids. Adding a pinch of high-quality sea salt (see recommendations on page 15) will restore trace minerals and electrolytes lost on long runs. Sip this instead of a neon blue sports drink!

2 cups unfiltered apple juice (fresh-pressed if you can get it)

1 cup filtered water

2 cinnamon sticks

1-inch knob fresh ginger, peeled and grated (for a subtler ginger flavor, slice it instead)

⅛ teaspoon fine sea salt

1. In a medium saucepan or a large teapot, combine the apple juice, water, cinnamon, ginger, and salt. Bring to a boil, then reduce heat to low. Simmer, covered, for 15 minutes.

2. Carefully pour the hot cider through a fine mesh sieve into 2 mugs and garnish each mug with one of the cinnamon sticks.

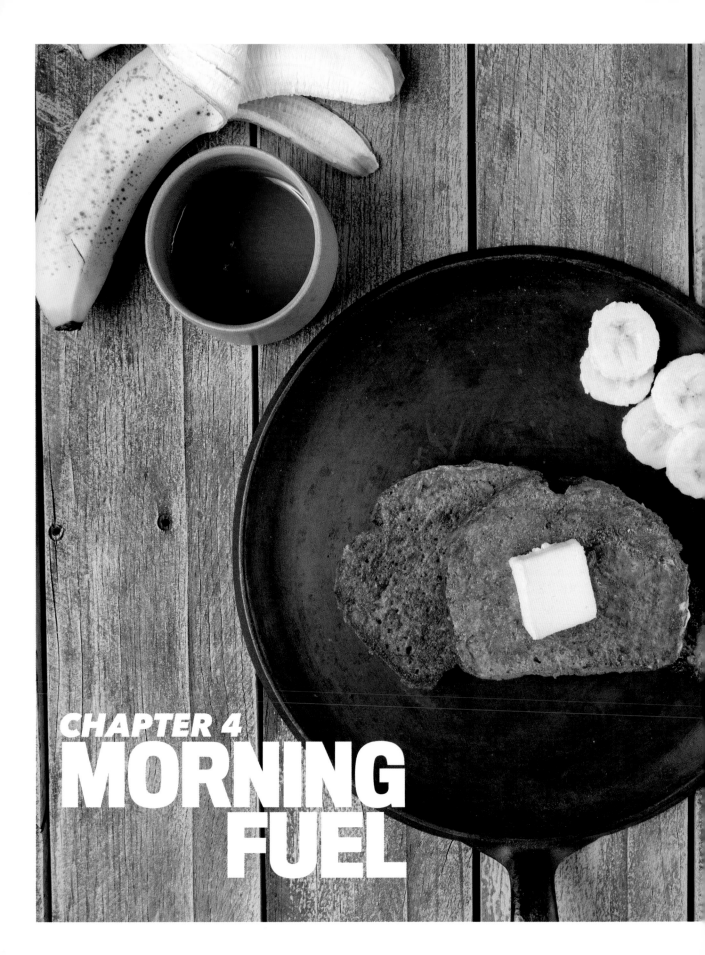

CHAPTER 4
MORNING
FUEL

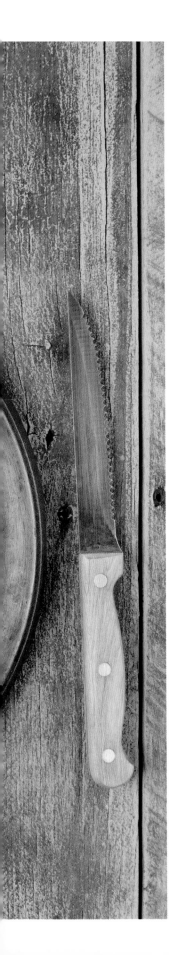

SUPERHERO MUFFINS

MAKES 12 MUFFINS

for a long Sunday run

If you have a high-powered blender, you can grind your own almond flour. For 2 cups of almond flour, pulse 10 ounces of whole raw almonds on high speed until finely ground.

Keep a batch in the freezer for a sweet grab-'n-run breakfast. Simply defrost on low power in the microwave.

These muffins were designed for superheroes like you. They're packed full of veggies and sweetened with maple syrup instead of refined sugar. In addition, almond meal and whole grain oats replace nutrient-stripped white flour. These are Shalane's go-to muffins—nourishing and sweetly satisfying for an easy grab-'n-run breakfast.

And don't fear the butter. Fueling up with healthy fats is a great way to start your day. Fat helps transport important vitamins throughout your hardworking body and will help keep you satisfied longer.

As a bonus, these muffins are gluten-free.

2 cups almond meal

1 cup old-fashioned rolled oats (gluten-free if sensitive)

2 teaspoons ground cinnamon

½ teaspoon ground nutmeg

1 teaspoon baking soda

½ teaspoon fine sea salt

½ cup chopped walnuts (optional)

½ cup raisins, chopped dates, or chocolate chips (optional)

3 eggs, beaten

1 cup grated zucchini (about 1 zucchini)

1 cup grated carrots (about 2 carrots)

6 tablespoons unsalted butter, melted

½ cup dark amber maple syrup

1 teaspoon vanilla extract

1. Position a rack in the center of the oven. Preheat the oven to 350°F. Line a 12-cup standard muffin tin with paper muffin cups.

2. In a large bowl, combine the almond meal, oats, cinnamon, nutmeg, baking soda, salt, and walnuts, raisins, dates, or chocolate chips (if using).

3. In a separate bowl, mix together the eggs, zucchini, carrots, butter, maple syrup, and vanilla. Add to the dry ingredients, mixing until just combined. The batter will be thick.

4. Spoon the batter into the muffin cups, filling each to the brim. Bake until the muffins are nicely browned on top and a toothpick inserted in the center of a muffin comes out clean, 25 to 35 minutes.

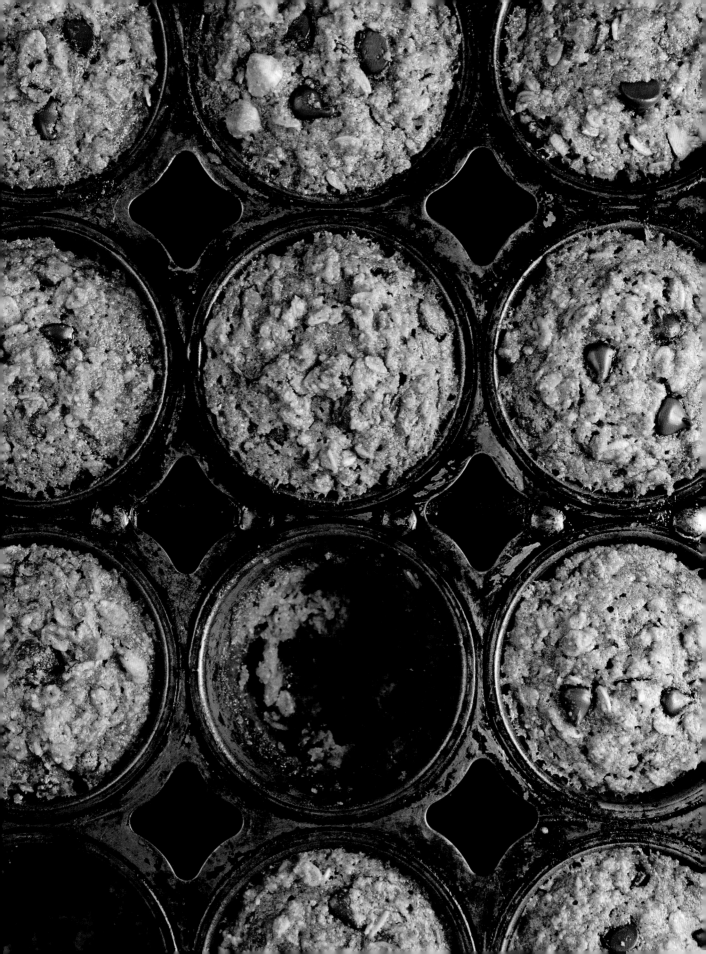

TEFF PUMPKIN PANCAKES WITH CURRANTS

MAKES 35 3-INCH PANCAKES

for postrace nourishment

We snooped around to see what Shalane's competition eats and discovered the nutritional powerhouse that is teff. An ancient East African cereal grass, teff has been a staple of Ethiopian cuisine for thousands of years. With all the running prowess coming out of Ethiopia, we couldn't help but explore the magic of this tiny grain.

Unlike most other flours, when teff is milled, the germ and bran are left intact. Our philosophy that the whole is greater than the sum of its parts definitely applies here. Teff flour is high in protein, fiber, calcium, magnesium, iron, zinc, and vitamin B_6—so move over, quinoa! It was a no-brainer to bring this wonder grain into Shalane's kitchen, and her first request was pancakes. A little pumpkin purée and holiday spice turned these nutty-tasting pancakes into a stack worthy of a postrace celebratory brunch.

For a fluffier stack, make the batter the night before to give the whole grains chance to soften. Store batter covered in the fridge. In the morning, lightly stir the batter to prevent popping all the air pockets.

This recipe makes a large stack of pancakes. Allow pancakes to cool completely prior to storing in the fridge or freezer. To reheat, simply pop individual pancakes in the toaster. It will taste light-years better than a frozen, store-bought waffle and be far healthier!

1½ cups teff flour (make sure the bag says "flour")

1 tablespoon baking powder

1 tablespoon pumpkin pie spice

1 teaspoon ground cinnamon

½ teaspoon fine sea salt

2 eggs, lightly beaten

1 cup canned pumpkin puree

1¾ cups unsweetened almond milk or other milk of choice

½ cup plain whole milk yogurt

2 tablespoons honey

½ cup currants or raisins

Safflower oil or other neutral, high-heat oil, for brushing the pan

1. In a large bowl, whisk together the teff flour, baking powder, pumpkin pie spice, cinnamon, and salt.

2. In a separate bowl, whisk together the eggs, pumpkin, milk, yogurt, and honey. Pour over the dry mixture and stir until just combined.

3. Fold in the currants or raisins. For best results, allow the batter to rest overnight in the fridge (see explanation above).

4. Heat a stovetop griddle or cast-iron skillet over medium-low heat. Use a brush or paper towel to lightly coat the pan with the oil. (Too much oil will cause burning.)

5. Ladle a heaping tablespoon of batter into the hot pan. Pour additional pancakes, leaving enough space between them for easy flipping. Cook the pancakes on one side until the bottoms start to brown, 1½ to 2 minutes. Using a metal spatula, flip the pancakes over and cook on the other side until nicely browned and cooked through, 1½ to 2 minutes. Continue with the remaining batter, brushing the pan with more oil, if needed.

6. Serve immediately with a pat of butter and a drizzle of maple syrup, or slather on some Coffee-Vanilla Peanut Butter (page 205). Cool leftovers completely before storing in the freezer.

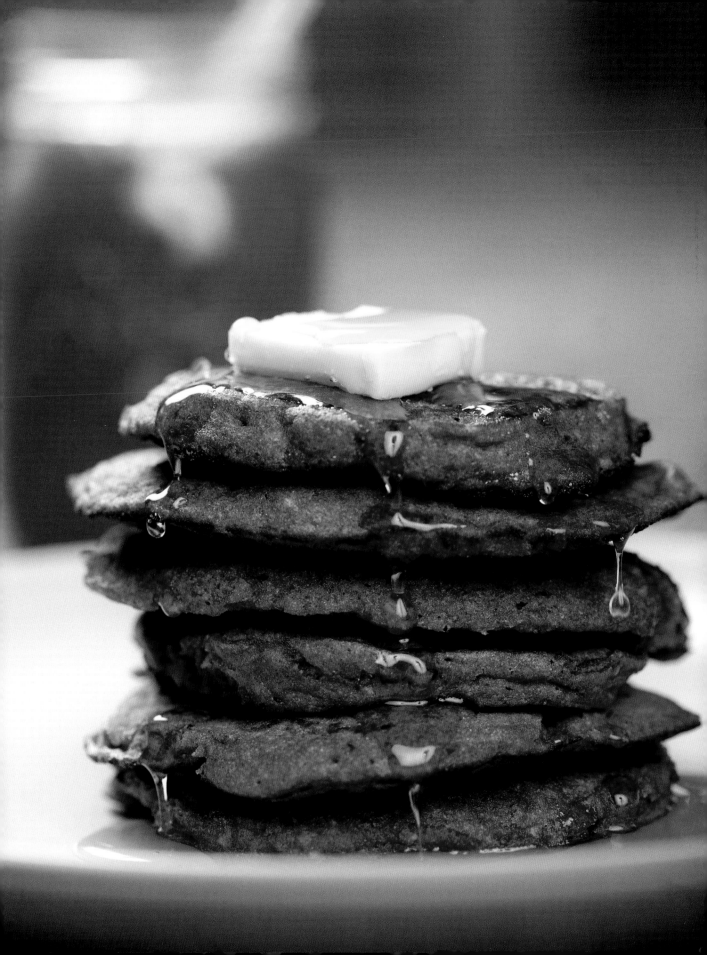

SWISS MUESLI BOWL

SERVES 2

for staying power

Shalane and Elyse share a joint love of Switzerland and especially the Swiss Alps. We were lucky enough to backpack together through this insanely beautiful country during summer break after our junior year of college. Then we were both doubly lucky and got to live in Switzerland for a while—Shalane for high-altitude training in St. Moritz, and Elyse for an international marketing job in Geneva.

Bircher Muesli, named after Maximilian Bircher-Benner, the Swiss doctor who developed this raw oat bowl for his patients in early 1900, stands out as the clear breakfast winner from our time spent in Switzerland. It's traditionally made with heavy cream, but to make it easier to digest, we've swapped in almond milk.

To give your morning extra oomph, add a spoonful of chia seeds. Sounds like hippy food, but those tiny seeds have serious staying power. After all, they were a staple food for Aztec warriors in the 16th century.

1 cup old-fashioned rolled oats (gluten-free if sensitive)

¾ cup unsweetened almond milk or other milk of choice (Homemade Hazelnut Milk, page 34)

¾ cup plain whole milk yogurt

2 teaspoons honey

1 teaspoon ground cinnamon

Dash of vanilla extract (optional)

Pinch of fine sea salt

1 Granny Smith apple, unpeeled, grated

Optional toppings: fresh berries, chia seeds or sunflower seeds, chopped walnuts or pecans, toasted coconut flakes, chopped dates or other dried fruit

1. In a medium bowl, combine the oats, milk, yogurt, honey, cinnamon, vanilla (if using), and salt. Cover and allow to soak for at least 1 hour or refrigerate overnight.

2. Stir in the apple and add more milk, if too thick.

3. Divide between 2 bowls, then stir in any assortment of toppings (if desired). We love to top ours with fresh berries.

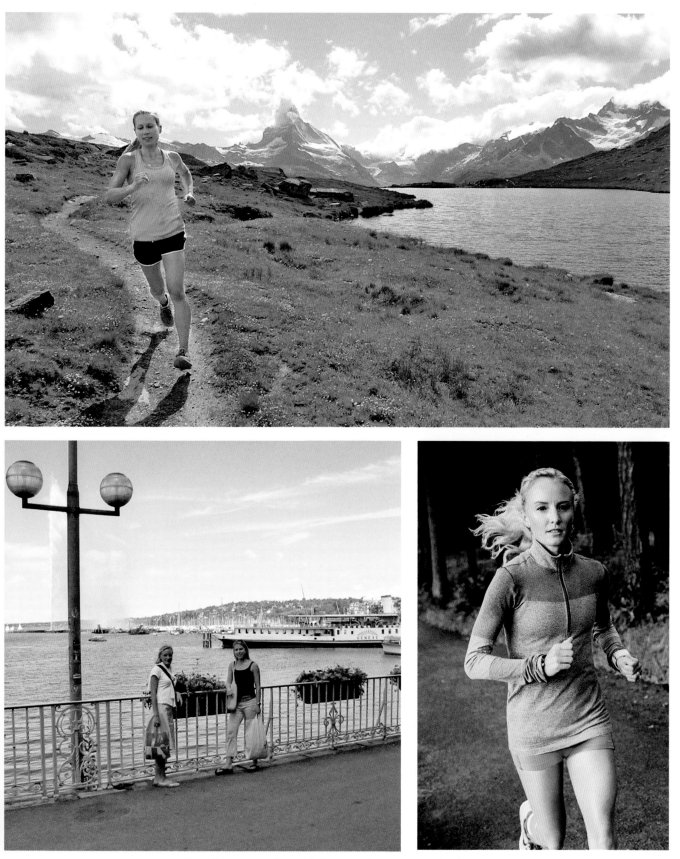

Top: Elyse running beneath the Matterhorn in Switzerland in 2011.
Bottom left: Shalane and Elyse together in Geneva during a college backpacking trip in 2003.

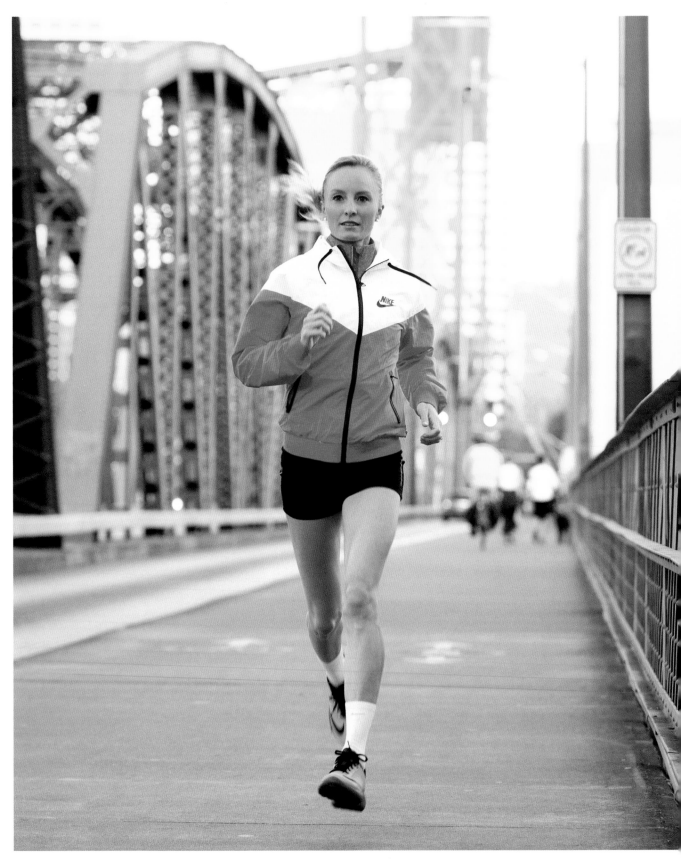

Shalane running across the Hawthorne Bridge in Portland, Oregon.

MAKE-AHEAD BREAKFAST BURRITOS

MAKES 6 BURRITOS

for a hearty postrun breakfast

If you get as hungry as we do after a morning run, then this is the breakfast to have ready and waiting when you walk back in the door. We lived on burritos during our college days, and we can't seem to kick the craving.

Our homemade breakfast burritos are designed to nourish a hungry runner. They're a protein-packed powerhouse, thanks to the incredible combo of eggs and beans. They're also loaded with fiber, calcium, and iron. Seek out a good brand of whole grain tortillas with a short list of ingredients and you'll be one step ahead of the competition.

The best part about this recipe is that it makes enough for you to devour one now and freeze five for future postrun breakfasts (or dinners!). See reheating instructions at the end of this recipe. To keep your body fueled on whole foods, keep your freezer stocked with homemade meals that can be reheated in minutes.

1 tablespoon olive oil

1 bag (6 ounces) baby spinach (about 4 packed cups)

10 eggs, beaten

½ teaspoon fine sea salt

¼ teaspoon freshly ground black pepper

6 burrito-size whole grain tortillas (about 10 inches)

1½ cups grated Gruyere or other favorite cheese

1½ cups Spicy Black Beans (page 162) or 1 can (15 ounces) chili beans

1. Heat the oil in a large nonstick skillet (eggs are the one dish we cook in a nonstick pan) over medium heat. Add the spinach and cook until just wilted. Add the eggs, salt, and pepper and cook, stirring continuously, until scrambled. Remove from the heat.

2. Place each tortilla on a 12 x 12-inch sheet of aluminum foil and sprinkle with ¼ cup of the cheese. Divide the egg-spinach mixture among the 6 tortillas, placing in a strip down the center of the wrap. Top each with ¼ cup of the beans.

3. Roll up each tortilla like a burrito by folding in the tops and bottoms, and wrap tightly in the foil. Place together in a gallon-size freezer bag and freeze for up to 2 months.

4. To reheat, unwrap from the foil, place on a microwaveable plate, and microwave on high for 2 to 3 minutes, rotating after 1 minute, until warm in the center.

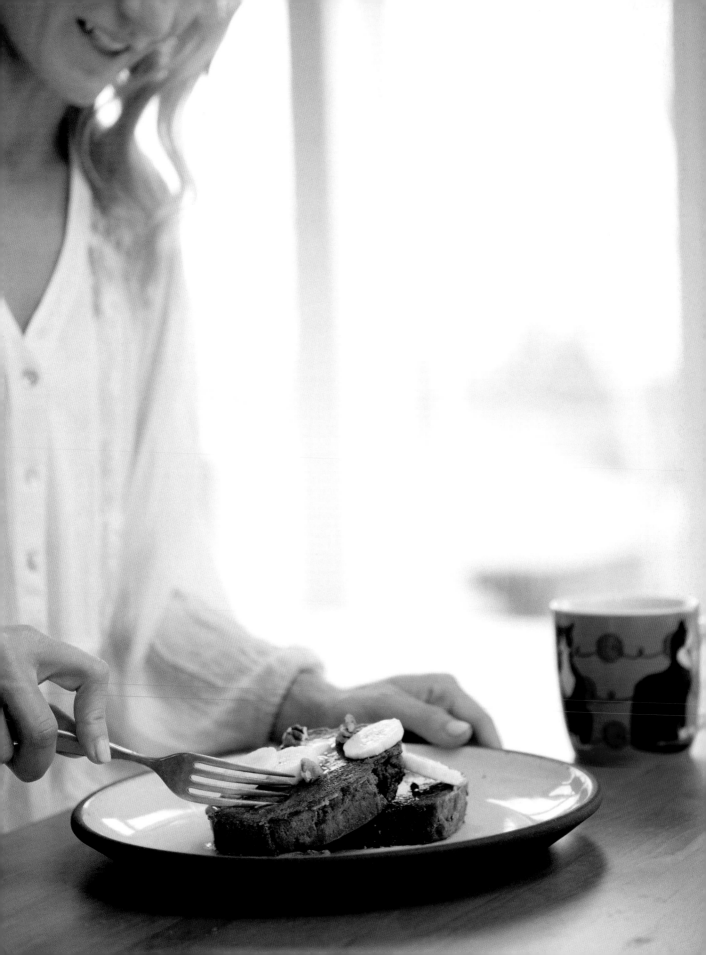

BANANA BREAD FRENCH TOAST

SERVES 4

for memorable mornings

We're not sure why french toast doesn't get as much limelight as pancakes and waffles—your favorite bread dipped in eggs and fried until golden? It doesn't get much better than that. According to recipe tester Amy Wolff, "One has not lived until they have had Banana Bread French Toast."

A childhood-cherished breakfast of Elyse's was french toast made with thick slices of homemade banana bread. When Shalane heard about this breakfast treat, she had to try it, so we re-created Elyse's long-lost family recipe.

If you made a loaf of our Spelt Banana Bread (page 183), then we highly recommend hiding half of the loaf so that when the weekend rolls around, you can transform it into a memorable brunch. Banana bread that is a couple of days old works best since it will hold together better. This recipe is also fabulous made with our Ginger-Molasses Quick Bread (page 182). For a more savory french toast, your favorite whole grain bread can be swapped in.

---

4 eggs

¼ cup unsweetened almond milk or other milk of choice (Homemade Hazelnut Milk, page 34)

½ teaspoon ground cinnamon

½ teaspoon almond extract

⅛ teaspoon fine sea salt

Pinch of ground nutmeg (optional)

Twist of freshly ground black pepper

2 tablespoons butter

8 1-inch-thick slices Spelt Banana Bread (page 183) or other bread of choice

Optional toppings: coarse sea salt, sliced bananas, maple syrup

1. In an 8 x 8-inch baking dish or a flat-bottomed bowl, whisk together the eggs, milk, cinnamon, almond extract, salt, nutmeg (if using), and pepper.

2. Melt 1 tablespoon of the butter in a large skillet over medium-high heat. Dip each slice of bread in the egg mixture, flipping to coat both sides, and set on a plate.

3. Place 4 of the slices in the skillet, pouring a little extra egg mixture over top. Fry until golden brown, 1 to 2 minutes. Use a spatula to carefully flip each slice, and repeat on the second side. If the butter in the pan begins to burn, use a folded paper towel to carefully wipe it out, add another tablespoon of butter, and repeat with the remaining 4 slices.

4. Serve immediately topped with a sprinkle of coarse sea salt, banana slices, and/or a drizzle of maple syrup (if desired).

ON-THE-RUN FRITTATA MUFFINS

MAKES 12 MUFFINS

for a satisfying breakfast-to-go

Experiment with mixing in different seasonal veggies. Leftover roasted root veggies are unbeatable in a frittata. Simply substitute 3 cups diced roasted vegetables for the onion, red pepper, sweet potato, and kale. See page 29 for tips on roasting roots.

When we announced on social media that we were writing this cookbook, we were over-the-moon thrilled by the enthusiasm we received from the running community. Immediately we started receiving inspiring ideas. One of the most common requests was for easy, healthy breakfast options.

Stephanie Kliethermes requested "breakfast options that can be made on Sundays and used the rest of the week at work." Since eggs are a fabulous way for runners to start their day, we decided to come up with an *egg-cellent* breakfast that can be made in advance and packed to go. And so these veggie-loaded, protein-packed Frittata Muffins were born (thanks, Stephanie!).

We now keep these little egg muffins stored in our freezers for time-crunched hungry mornings (that's every morning!).

9 eggs

½ cup crumbled feta or other favorite cheese

¼ cup plain whole milk yogurt

¼ teaspoon freshly ground black pepper

2 tablespoons extra-virgin olive oil

1 yellow onion, finely chopped

1 red bell pepper, seeded and finely chopped

1 sweet potato (12 ounces), unpeeled, cut into ½-inch cubes

¼ teaspoon fine sea salt

2 cups loosely packed, chopped kale, stems removed

1. Preheat the oven to 325°F. Line a standard 12-cup muffin pan with foil muffin cups (for easier cleanup) or grease the pan with butter.

2. In a large bowl, whisk together the eggs, cheese, yogurt, and pepper.

3. Heat the oil in a large skillet over medium heat. Add the onion, red bell pepper, sweet potato, and salt and cook, stirring occasionally, until lightly browned (the potatoes won't be cooked through), about 10 minutes. Add the veggies to the egg mixture.

4. In the same skillet, cook the kale, stirring constantly, just until wilted, about 3 minutes. Add the kale to the egg mixture.

5. Spoon the mixture into the muffin cups, filling each one even to the brim. Bake in the center of the oven until the eggs have set and the tops are golden, 35 to 40 minutes.

6. Transfer the muffins to a plate for serving. Or cool completely and store in an airtight container in the fridge for up to 5 days or in the freezer for up to 1 month.

7. To reheat frozen frittata muffins, remove the foil muffin cup and place on a microwaveable dish. Heat on low for 1½ to 2 minutes, just until warm.

RACE DAY OATMEAL

SERVES 1

for easily digested energy

🕐 When you're on the road for a race, simply use boiling water from an electric tea kettle to make this breakfast in less than 5 minutes.

🏅 For slower mornings, use steel-cut oats instead of instant oats and cook over the stovetop according to package directions. Then stir in the toppings.

The story behind this recipe runs deep. For more than 8 years, this has been Shalane's go-to breakfast before all her hard workouts and races. Running her first marathon ever in NYC, rocking the marathon at the London Olympics, running the fastest time ever by an American woman at the Boston Marathon—all such performances were powered by this recipe.

As a whole foods chef, Elyse was at first doubtful about using instant oats and a microwave and calling it breakfast. Her first trial resulted in a thick, globby mess that her then 9-month-old daughter, Lily, completely refused. Elyse called Shalane into her kitchen for damage control, and at last we got the recipe drafted up exactly how Shalane prepares it.

Shalane likes to add the banana prior to microwaving for a creamy texture and fresh-baked banana bread flavor. Being slightly superstitious and true to her Irish roots, Shalane brings along her favorite brand of oats, McCann's Quick Cooking Irish Oatmeal, whenever she's on the road.

½ cup instant oats (gluten-free if sensitive)

1 banana, sliced

Pinch of sea salt

¼ cup almond milk or other milk of choice (Homemade Hazelnut Milk, page 34)

Walnuts or almond butter

Raisins or fresh berries

Ground cinnamon

Honey (optional)

Combine the oats, banana, salt, and ¾ cup water in a microwave-able bowl. Microwave on high power for 1 to 2 minutes, or until thickened. Mash the banana slightly and stir in the milk. Stir in the walnuts or almond butter and raisins or berries to taste. Top with a sprinkle of cinnamon and a drizzle of honey if desired.

GINGER-MOLASSES GRANOLA

MAKES 8 CUPS (16 SERVINGS)

for nourished snacking

A hearty granola packed with oats and seeds is a must for athletes, but the expensive store-bought stuff with endless health claims plastered on the colorful packages is loaded with sugar. Our ginger-spiked granola is lightly sweetened with blackstrap molasses, the sticky good stuff that's left behind after sugarcane is refined. That makes it high in minerals, including potassium, calcium, iron, and magnesium—minerals many athletes don't get enough of.

Be warned: If you share your homemade granola with friends and family, they'll be asking you to make it time and again.

---

3 cups old-fashioned rolled oats (gluten-free if sensitive)

1 cup finely shredded unsweetened dried coconut

½ cup shelled pumpkin seeds

½ cup sunflower seeds

½ cup raisins or chopped dried fruit

2 teaspoons ground ginger

2 teaspoons ground cinnamon

½ teaspoon fine sea salt

⅓ cup virgin coconut oil

¼ cup honey

¼ cup blackstrap molasses (darkest variety, which has a stronger flavor and more minerals than regular molasses)

1. Position a rack in the center of the oven. Preheat the oven to 275°F and line a rimmed baking sheet with parchment paper.

2. In a large mixing bowl, stir together the oats, coconut, pumpkin seeds, sunflower seeds, raisins or dried fruit, ginger, cinnamon, and salt.

3. In a small microwaveable bowl, stir together the coconut oil, honey, and molasses and microwave on low until slightly melted. Or melt in a small saucepan over low heat. Pour over the dry ingredients and stir until evenly combined.

4. Spread out in a thick layer on the baking sheet. Bake, gently stirring every 15 minutes, until lightly browned, 45 minutes. Granola will still be moist at the end of baking, but will morph into crunchy goodness once it cools completely.

5. Store in a glass jar with a lid at room temperature. Granola will stay fresh for several weeks and likely be devoured long before expiring.

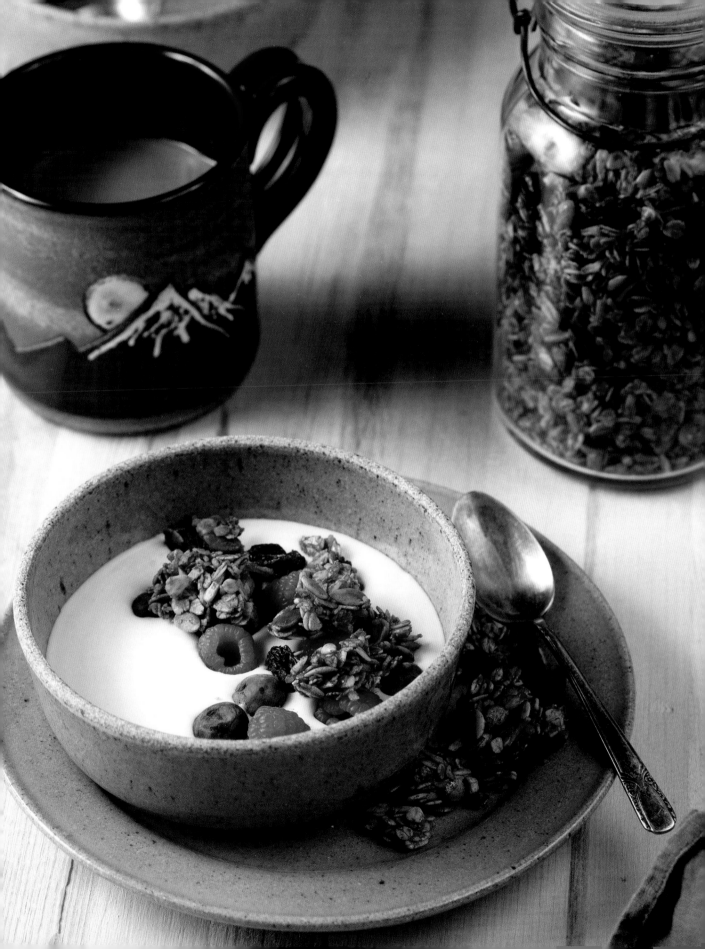

SWEET POTATO BREAKFAST COOKIES

MAKES 13 COOKIES

for fueling up on-the-go

NOTE: To make sweet potato puree, wrap 1 large (1 to 1½ pounds) orange-fleshed sweet potato (also called a yam) in foil. Bake at 400°F until tender, 45 to 60 minutes. Cool, remove the skin, and puree in a blender or food processor, or mash by hand with a fork until smooth. Puree can be made up to 5 days in advance and stored in the fridge. To save time, canned sweet potato puree can be found at many grocery stores.

Sweet potatoes in a cookie?! Yes, sweet potatoes in all their natural sweet glory are an incredible addition to baked goods. When devout distance trail runner and bakery owner Christine Mineart reached out to us to share this cookie recipe, we were immediately intrigued and baked up a batch right away.

Christine can be found running through the redwoods along the central California coast. After increasing her running intensity, Christine's health began to suffer until she turned to nourishing whole foods to better fuel her body. Now she is passionate about sharing her knowledge, and she opened Surf Muffins to bring her wholesome treats to her active community.

The next time you're baking sweet potatoes, throw an extra one in the oven, and when the weekend rolls around, get baking. We found ourselves loving these cookies for breakfast, they're that good and energizing. But they're also great any time of day.

---

3 cups old-fashioned rolled oats (gluten-free if sensitive)

1 cup almond flour or almond meal

1 tablespoon grated fresh ginger or 1 teaspoon ground

2 teaspoons ground cinnamon

½ teaspoon baking powder

½ teaspoon fine sea salt

1 cup orange-fleshed sweet potato (yam) puree (see note)

½ cup grade B maple syrup

½ cup coconut oil, melted

1 teaspoon vanilla extract

½ cup raisins

1. Preheat the oven to 350°F. Line a baking sheet with parchment paper.

2. In the bowl of a food processor or high-speed blender, pulse the oats 5 or 6 times, until roughly chopped. Place in a large mixing bowl and combine with the almond flour, ginger, cinnamon, baking powder, and salt.

3. In a separate bowl, whisk together the sweet potato puree, maple syrup, coconut oil, vanilla, and raisins until well combined. Fold into the oat mixture and stir until blended. The dough should be very thick.

4. Use a ¼ cup measuring cup to drop the batter onto the baking sheet. Space the cookies 1 inch apart and lightly press down on each one to slightly flatten.

5. Bake in the center of the oven until the bottoms are a deep golden brown, 25 to 30 minutes.

GIDDY-UP ENERGY BITES

MAKES 24 BITES

for preworkout energy

NOTE: To toast coconut, preheat the oven to 350°F and spread the dried coconut out on a baking sheet. Bake until golden, 4 to 5 minutes, stirring halfway through (keep a close eye on it to prevent burning).

Most packaged energy bars are full of highly processed sweeteners and a list of unpronounceable ingredients. These bars also come with a steep price tag. Our Giddy-Up Energy Bites skip the nonsense and get down to business.

Devour one (or three!) and you'll have the energy to outrun a bull. We say that because (and this is a little secret) Shalane was quite the fan of the North Carolina rodeo during our Tar Heel days. Once a year, we got decked out in our finest cowgirl gear and made our way to the fairgrounds for a night of good ole-fashioned rodeo fun. We could have used an energy bite like this to make our workout the morning after a little less painful.

12 large Medjool dates, pitted

1 cup dried unsweetened cherries

1 cup raw chopped walnuts

¼ cup unsalted almond butter (if salted, skip the salt below)

1 tablespoon unsweetened cocoa powder

2 tablespoons finely ground coffee beans (grind fresh)

¼ teaspoon fine sea salt

½ cup shredded unsweetened dried coconut, toasted (see note)

1. In a food processor, combine the dates, cherries, walnuts, almond butter, cocoa powder, coffee, and salt. Pulse a few times to chop the ingredients, and then process on high speed for 1 to 2 minutes, stopping once or twice to scrape down the sides of the bowl and beneath the blade with a spatula. Process until the ingredients begin to clump together.

2. Empty the contents of the food processor into a medium bowl. Use your hands to shape the mixture into 24 walnut-size balls and roll each ball in the coconut. Store in an airtight container for up to 1 month or in the freezer for up to 6 months.

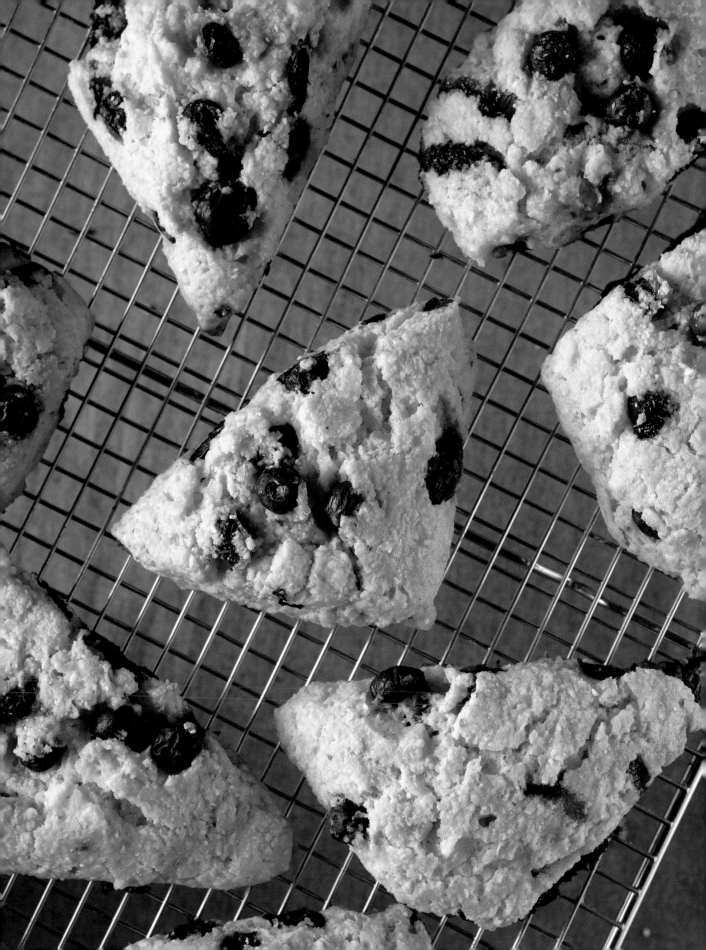

BLUEBERRY-LEMON CORNMEAL SCONES

MAKES 10 SCONES

for the love of brunch

Breakfast is our favorite meal of the day, especially when it's served after a long Sunday run. You walk in the door feeling accomplished, happy, and hungry. What better way to celebrate than with eggs, a basket of scones, and a mug of coffee (Shalane's a.m. drink of choice) or our Runners' Recovery Iced Tea (page 36).

These flaky, buttery scones satisfy our postrun cravings on every level. We love the texture and natural sweetness of the stone-ground cornmeal, enhanced by the blueberries and lemon zest.

Don't squawk at the amount of butter. Butter (from grass-fed cows) does the body good. Don't believe us? Learn more on page 17.

---

1 cup stone-ground cornmeal

1 cup all-purpose flour

¼ cup coconut sugar or other granulated sugar

2 teaspoons baking powder

½ teaspoon fine sea salt

1 stick (8 tablespoons) cold unsalted butter, cut into cubes

2 eggs

⅓ cup whole milk Greek yogurt

1 teaspoon vanilla extract

Finely grated zest of 2 lemons

1 cup frozen blueberries

1. Position a rack in the middle of the oven. Preheat the oven to 350°F. Line a baking sheet with parchment paper.

2. In a large mixing bowl, whisk together the cornmeal, flour, sugar, baking powder, and salt.

3. Using a pastry blender or your fingers, work the butter into the flour mixture until it's the size of peas.

4. In a separate bowl, whisk together the eggs, yogurt, vanilla, and lemon zest. Add to the dry ingredients and stir just until combined. Fold in the blueberries. The dough will be thick and sticky.

5. Flour a clean work surface and roll the dough into a semi-flattened log, about 2 inches in diameter. Cut the log into 10 triangles and place 2 inches apart on the baking sheet. Don't want to bother with a rolling pin? Simply drop the batter in large spoonfuls onto the baking sheet. Bake until lightly browned on the bottoms, 15 to 20 minutes. Transfer to a rack to cool.

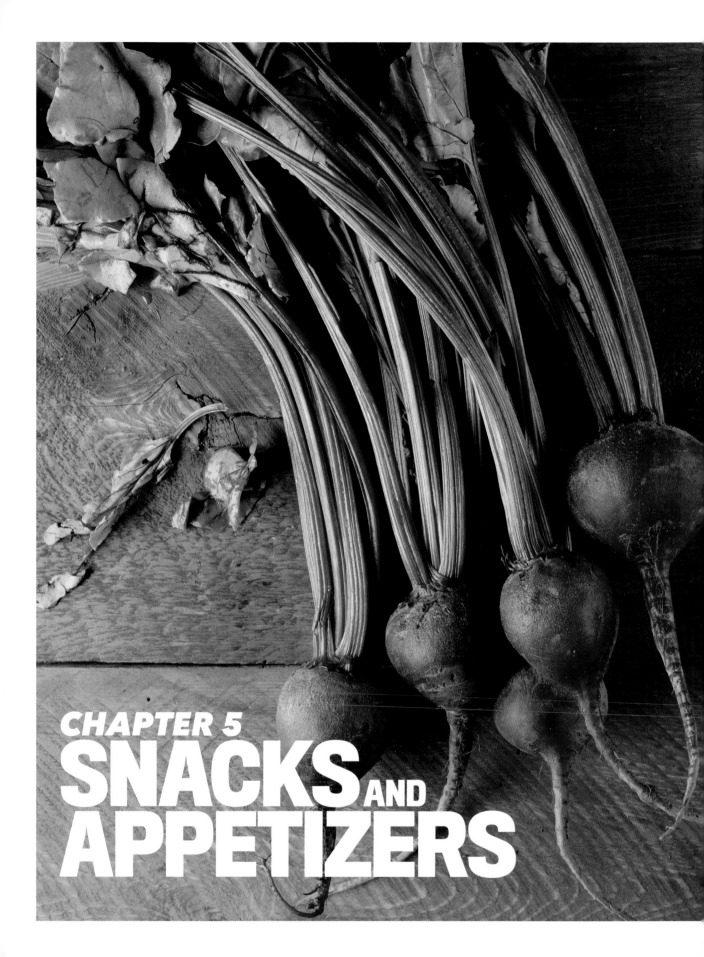

CHAPTER 5
SNACKS AND APPETIZERS

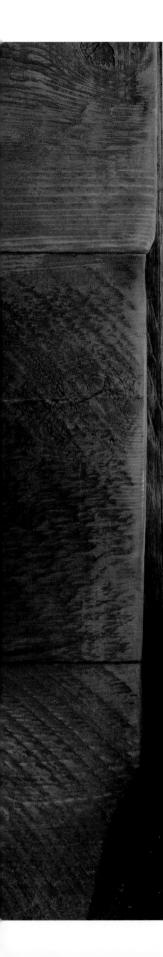

26.2 TRAIL MIX

SERVES 2

for energizing life's adventures

For hiking, camping trips, road trips, and long flights, we tote along a bag of trail mix filled with crunchy, energizing favorites.

Since ready-made trail mixes are loaded with refined sugar (a serving of yogurt-covered raisins or dried cranberries has more sugar than a candy bar), we bring to you 26.2 options to create a healthier trail mix. (The .2 is a sprinkle of cinnamon and sea salt!) Mix and match to your heart's content, or go wild and add all 26.2 ingredients.

NUTS

Pecans

Walnuts

Peanuts

Hazelnuts

Almonds

Cashews

Pistachios

SEEDS

Sunflower seeds

Pumpkin seeds

Hemp seeds

Sesame seeds

DRIED FRUIT

Date pieces

Raisins

Figs

Banana Chews (page 64)

Dried apricots (unsulfured)

Dried apples

Coconut flakes

OTHER

Pretzels

Popcorn

Wasabi peas

Sesame sticks

Ginger-Molasses Granola
(page 54)

Puffed rice

Dark chocolate chips

Cacao nibs

.2

Fine sea salt and cinnamon
(optional)

1. In a gallon-size freezer bag, combine any assortment of the listed ingredients. Add a sprinkle of salt and cinnamon (if desired). Close the bag, shake it up, then divide into snack-size bags for grab-'n-run convenience.

2. If the nuts are raw, we prefer to toast them (see Tip below) or soak them overnight and then dehydrate them (overnight in an oven at 150°F) prior to adding them to the trail mix.

TIP

To keep things crunchy, store the dried fruit separate from the rest of the mix and add in just before traveling.

TOASTING NUTS AND SEEDS

Seeds and small amounts of nuts can be toasted in a dry skillet over medium heat until fragrant. Larger batches of nuts should be toasted in the oven at 350°F, stirring every 4 minutes, for 8 to 12 minutes, depending on the type of nut.

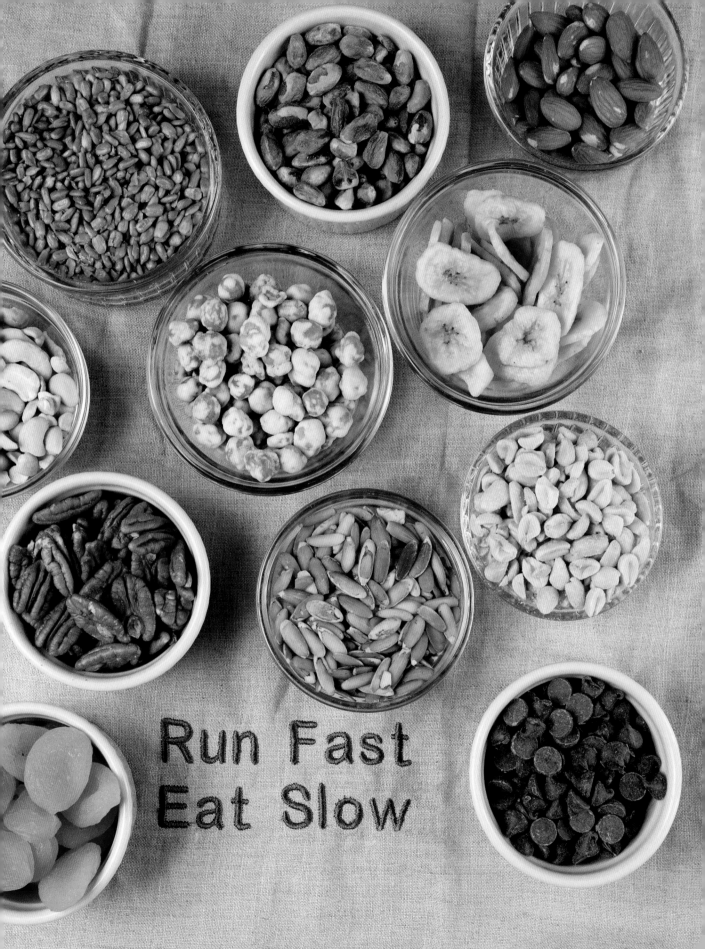

Run Fast
Eat Slow

BANANA CHEWS

MAKES ABOUT 80 CHEWS

for energy on the run

Bring a small bag along on your next long training run or toss into our 26.2 Trail Mix (page 62) for the perfect hiking companion.

One of the questions Shalane's fans ask most frequently is, "What do you eat during marathons?" The answer is nothing. Shalane prefers to take in only fluids (sports drink and water), but then again she's only on the marathon course for 2 hours and 22 minutes! For us mere mortals, who are out on the course much longer, we may find ourselves crashing without an extra energy boost.

Since we aren't fans of the artificial and overly sweet gel packets and gummies, we created these sweet little energizing banana chews that are highly portable. Bananas are naturally high in fructose and glucose, providing quick and balanced energy, and are a fantastic source of electrolytes. Our addicting chews have everything your hardworking body needs and nothing synthesized in a lab.

Also, unlike store-bought banana chips that are deep-fried and often coated in sugar, our banana chews are lightly brushed with a small amount of coconut oil and dusted with cinnamon and sea salt.

Be sure to test out any food and drink that you plan on consuming during race day well in advance.

---

2 tablespoons coconut oil, melted

1 tablespoon lemon juice

1 teaspoon ground cinnamon

¼ teaspoon fine sea salt

3 ripe bananas, peeled and sliced ⅛ inch thick

1. Preheat the oven to 250°F. Line a baking sheet with parchment paper and brush it with about 1 tablespoon of the coconut oil (a silicone basting brush works great).

2. In a small bowl, combine the remaining 1 tablespoon coconut oil, the lemon juice, cinnamon, and salt.

3. Spread out the bananas evenly on the baking sheet and brush each slice with the lemon mixture.

4. Bake in the center of the oven for 2 hours. After 1 hour, remove from the oven. Use tongs to flip each banana slice and return them to the oven.

5. Place the baking sheet on a wire rack to cool completely before storing in a mason jar or airtight container for up to 1 month.

WILDWOOD HAZELNUTS

MAKES 2 CUPS

for a nourishing crunch

We named these adventurous hazelnuts after Wildwood Trail, our favorite 30-mile running trail in Portland's Forest Park. Not to brag, but did you know our city has the nation's largest urban forest? Oh, and that Oregon produces 99 percent of the US crop of hazelnuts? Yes, we feel pretty lucky to call Portland home.

These salty-sweet-spicy nuts are designed to satisfy all your snack-attack cravings. And they'll work hard for you—hazelnuts are rich in manganese (a vital nutrient for strong bones), folate (an essential vitamin for cardiovascular health), and copper (a mineral needed for proper iron absorption).

Snacking on a few of these well-spiced nuts before dinner will get your digestive juices flowing. They're also fabulous on top of salads, especially our Oregon Summer Salad with Grilled Salmon (page 82), Strawberry-Arugula Kamut Salad (page 81), or a simple green salad with goat cheese and roasted beets.

2 tablespoons butter

2 teaspoons ground cinnamon

½ teaspoon ground red pepper

2 tablespoons honey

¾ teaspoon fine sea salt

2 cups raw hazelnuts

1. Preheat the oven to 350°F. Line a baking sheet with parchment paper.

2. Melt the butter on medium-low in a medium skillet or saucepan. Add the cinnamon and pepper and cook until fragrant, stirring continuously, about 1 minute. Remove pan from the heat and stir in the honey and salt. Add the hazelnuts and stir to coat.

3. Spread the hazelnuts on the baking sheet and roast in the center of the oven for 15 minutes, stirring every 5 minutes.

4. Cool completely in a single layer, then break apart any clusters and transfer to a glass jar.

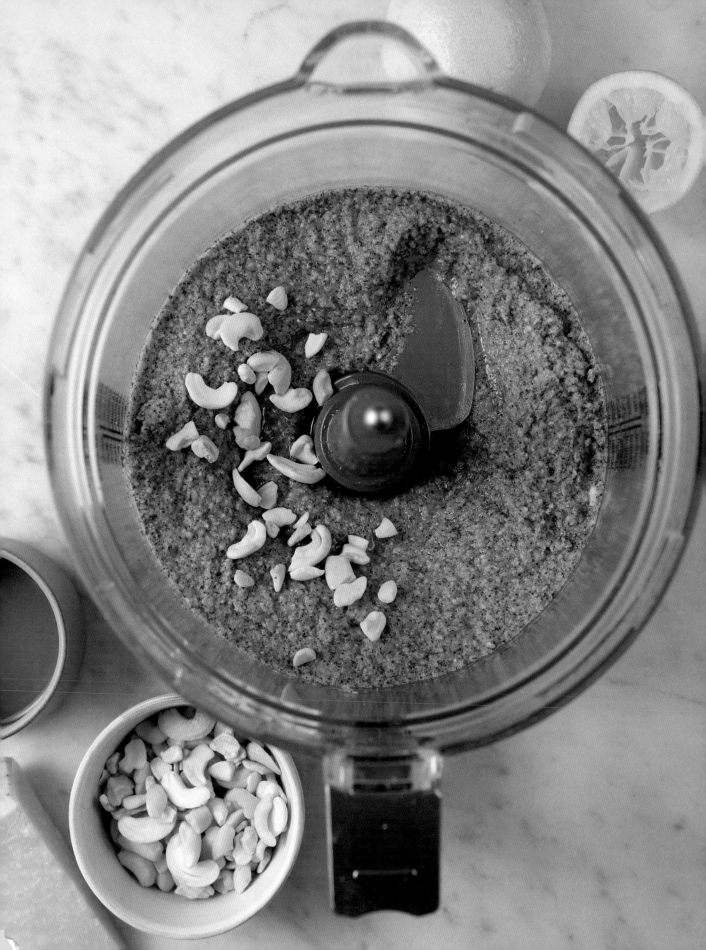

ARUGULA CASHEW PESTO

MAKES 2 CUPS

for digestion-enhancing flavor

Toss with Zucchini Pesto "Pasta" (page 122) and top with grilled salmon to make it a meal.

Save that expensive Parmesan rind and toss it into soups for a more flavorful broth. See our Hearty Minestrone with Spicy Sausage and Beans (page 107).

Arugula in pesto?! Yes, you read that correctly. Did you know arugula is a calcium-rich food? And that calcium, from whole food sources, is key to maintaining muscle function and bone health? (Stress fractures be gone!) With its vibrant, spicy flavor, arugula brings this pesto to life, making it the perfect accent to many dishes. Plus, the miso in this pesto will aid your digestion, the garlic will boost your immune system, and the nuts, Parmesan, and olive oil will provide you with necessary healthy fats.

We highly recommend making a double batch. (If you're like us, you'll be eating this stuff by the spoonful straight out of the jar!) Freezing what you don't use in an ice cube tray makes for easy weeknight meals. Toss this versatile pesto with your favorite pasta, roasted vegetables, or potatoes. It also is terrific spooned on top of grilled fish, chicken, and steak and can even replace marinara sauce on pizza (page 134).

A heads-up: You'll need a food processor or professional blender to make this recipe.

1 cup toasted cashews or walnuts (see "Toasting Nuts and Seeds" on page 62)

2 cups tightly packed arugula (or basil, beet greens, or turnip greens)

1¼ cups grated Parmesan cheese

1 or 2 cloves garlic

½ cup extra-virgin olive oil

2 teaspoons white miso paste

2 to 3 tablespoons lemon juice

1 teaspoon lemon zest

1. In a food processor or professional blender, combine the nuts, arugula (or basil, beet greens, or turnip greens), Parmesan, and garlic. Process until coarsely chopped. Add the oil, miso, lemon juice, and zest. Process until desired consistency is reached. We like our pesto slightly chunky.

2. Transfer to a container with a tight-fitting lid, and store in the refrigerator for up to 5 days or freeze for up to 3 months. (The pesto can be thinned to make a sauce. Simply add more olive oil, broth, or water.)

TIP

To make this recipe vegan and dairy-free, leave out the Parmesan and add 2 extra teaspoons of miso. Miso has a similar salty, umami flavor profile.

CROSTINI WITH CHÈVRE, FIGS, AND THYME

SERVES 5

for a sweet and savory appetizer

Crostini—grilled bread piled with any assortment of toppings—is a foolproof appetizer to serve to hungry guests. We can't tell you how many times we have served this variation topped with sweet and savory favorites! Come end of summer, we top the chèvre with fresh figs; when winter rolls around, we revert to ripe pear slices. Any time of year, a sprinkle of thyme and sea salt and a drizzle of honey will awaken all your taste buds just in time for dinner.

½ large baguette or 1 small baguette (about 1 foot), cut into ½-inch-thick slices

Extra-virgin olive oil, for drizzling

1 large clove garlic

1 package (4 ounces) natural chèvre (goat cheese)

4 or 5 fresh figs, sliced thin, or ½ ripe pear, sliced thin

Honey, for drizzling

1 tablespoon fresh thyme leaves

Coarse sea salt

1. Set the oven to broil with a rack on the upper shelf.

2. Place the baguette slices on a rimmed baking sheet and drizzle one side generously with oil. Place under the broiler and toast until lightly browned, about 1 minute. Watch carefully to prevent burning. Remove from the oven, flip each slice, and broil the second side for 30 seconds to 1 minute.

3. Rub one side of each crostini with the garlic and arrange on a platter. Top with a smear of chèvre, a fig (or pear) slice, a drizzle of honey, and a sprinkle of thyme and salt.

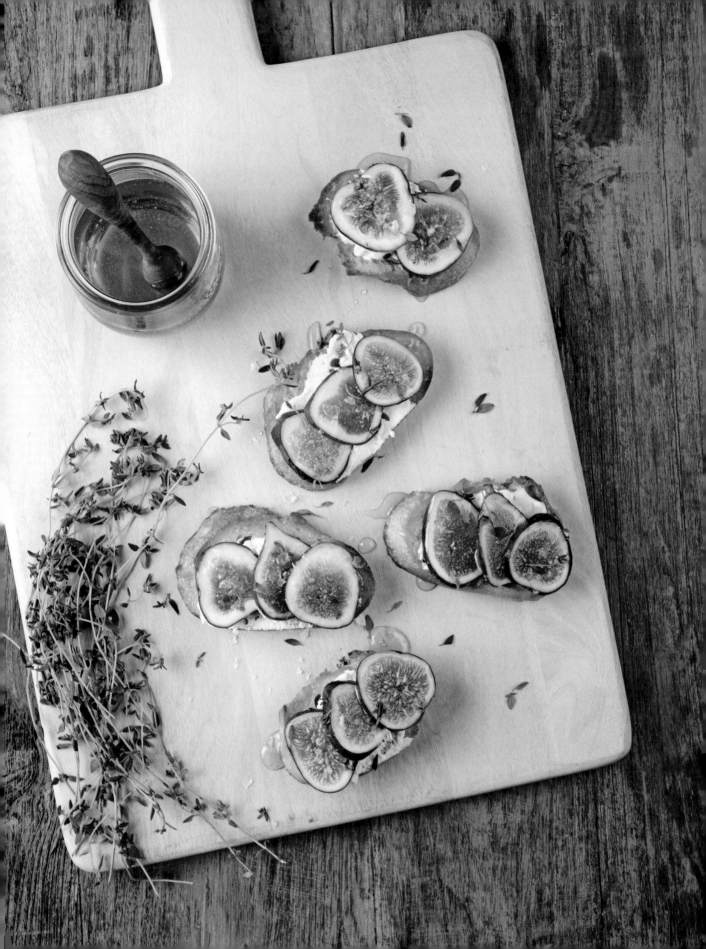

CHIPOTLE HUMMUS

MAKES 1¾ CUPS

for staving off hunger until dinner

Hummus is about the easiest thing to whip together when you have hungry guests arriving and dinner isn't quite ready. For this reason, we always keep cans of chickpeas stacked in our pantries. Once you get hooked on our homemade hummus, you'll discover that the store-bought stuff deserves to get left in the dust. It's seriously lacking in fresh flavor due to added preservatives.

If you like fiery flavor, our Chipotle Hummus will do the trick. (If earthy sweetness is more your style, turn the page for our Don't Get Beet Hummus.) All it takes is the addition of one chipotle pepper to add serious heat. Or remove the seeds from the peppers for a milder result. You'll need a food processor or high-speed blender to achieve creamy perfection.

1 can (15 ounces) chickpeas, rinsed and drained, or 1½ cups cooked

1 chipotle pepper in adobo sauce

2 tablespoons tahini

3 tablespoons fresh lemon juice (1 to 2 lemons)

¼ cup extra-virgin olive oil

½ teaspoon fine sea salt

1. In a food processor or high-speed blender, combine the chickpeas, chipotle pepper, tahini, lemon juice, oil, and salt. Blend on high until smooth, stopping as needed to scrape down the sides and underneath the blade with a rubber spatula. If too thick, thin by adding 1 tablespoon water at a time.

2. Transfer to a glass jar or bowl with a lid. Chill in the fridge until ready to serve. Serve with homemade Pita Chips with Oregano and Sea Salt (page 74) or tortilla chips and carrot sticks.

TIP

Freeze leftover chipotle peppers for future spicy shenanigans.

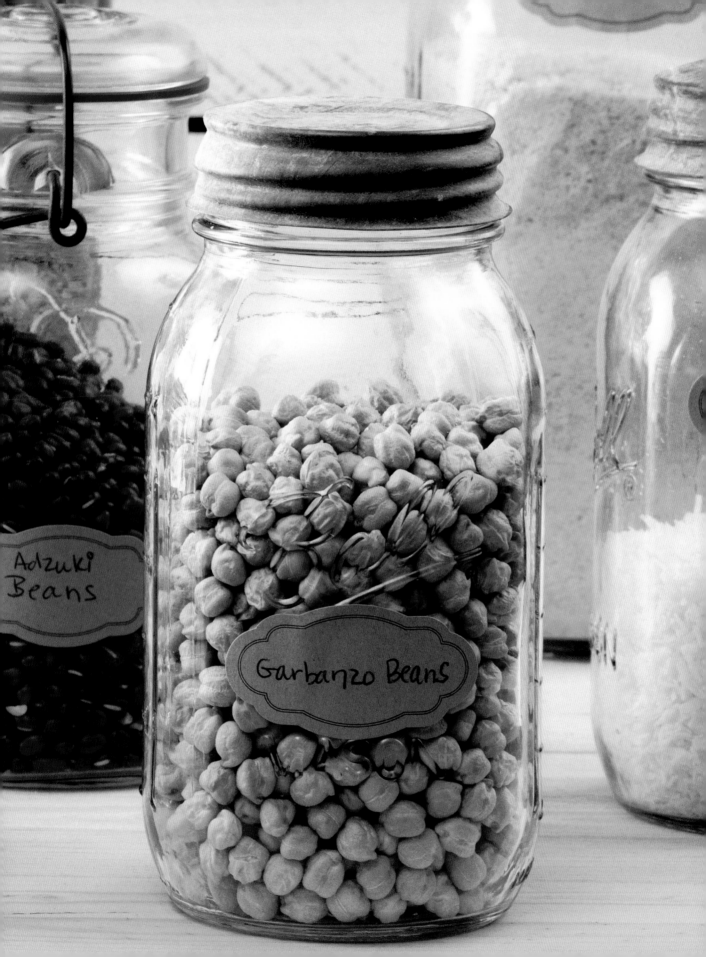

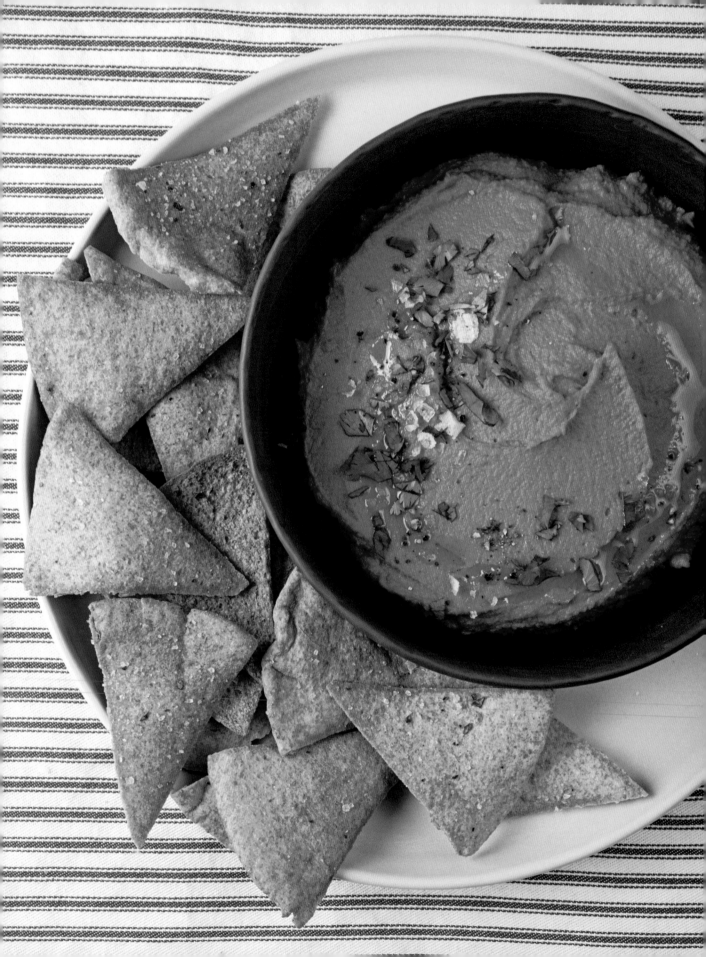

DON'T GET BEET HUMMUS

MAKES 2 CUPS

for impressing dinner guests

Don't toss those nutrient-rich beet greens! Use them in smoothies, stir-fries, or Arugula Cashew Pesto (page 67).

Use the leftovers as a vibrant alternative to marinara sauce on homemade pizza.

If you're still not making your own hummus from scratch (we told you why you need to join our hummus-making club on page 70), then this recipe will get you hooked. The color alone will lure your guests to the table. Then you can tell them your hummus is made with purple tulips—or let them in on the real secret.

Plan ahead and simply wrap a beet in foil and toss it in the oven with whatever else you're cooking. That way, when you want to make this hummus, you'll be ready!

1 can (15 ounces) chickpeas, rinsed and drained, or 1½ cups cooked

1 medium beet, roasted (see page 29), peeled, and quartered

1 clove garlic

2 tablespoons tahini

3 tablespoons fresh lemon juice

¼ cup extra-virgin olive oil

¾ teaspoon fine sea salt

Optional garnishes: chopped cilantro, flaky sea salt, olive oil

1. In a food processor or high-speed blender, combine the chickpeas, beet, garlic, tahini, lemon juice, olive oil, and salt. Process on high until smooth, stopping as needed to scrape down the sides and underneath the blade with a rubber spatula.

2. Transfer to a small serving bowl and garnish with chopped cilantro, flaky sea salt, and/or a drizzle of olive oil (if desired). Serve with Pita Chips with Oregano and Sea Salt (page 74), Crostini (page 68), or carrot sticks.

TIP

Tahini is made from ground sesame seeds and can be found near the nut butters in most grocery stores. Or buy hulled sesame seeds and grind your own (see page 204).

PITA CHIPS WITH OREGANO AND SEA SALT

SERVES 6

for a backyard BBQ

We were so in love with our Chipotle Hummus and Don't Get Beet Hummus (pages 70 and 73) that we needed to come up with a crunchy companion worthy of dipping.

Sure, you can go out and buy a bag of pita chips, but we know you'll like this version better. Experiment and create your own variation by adding different dried herbs and spices.

6 whole wheat pita breads (pocket style)

½ cup extra-virgin olive oil

1 teaspoon dried oregano

¾ teaspoon coarse sea salt

1. Preheat the oven to 300°F.

2. Run a knife along the edge of each pita to separate into 2 rounds. Use a silicone basting brush to brush both sides generously with the oil (alternatively you can drizzle the oil over top). Stack the rounds and slice each into 8 triangles (you'll get 16 chips per pita bread).

3. Spread the chips out on 2 rimmed baking sheets (some overlapping is fine). Sprinkle with the oregano and salt.

4. Bake on the center and lower racks of the oven until crisp, 20 minutes.

5. Cool, then store in a gallon-size resealable bag for up to 1 month.

6. You can also serve this with Avocado Cream (page 178).

ROASTED GARLIC

1 BULB

for endless inspiration

🕐 No need to run your oven for one lonely bulb of garlic. To save energy, plan ahead and pop the bulb in your oven with whatever else you're cooking. Simply adjust the cook time to longer or shorter if you're roasting at a lower or higher temp.

If you don't like garlic, then we need to have a little talk. Garlic has the ability to transform the mundane into greatness. For this reason alone, we champion garlic in a lot of our recipes. But there's more. Garlic is also an anti-inflammatory warrior and virus-fighting champion.

An entire bulb of garlic simply roasted with a drizzle of olive oil yields an irresistible, sweet, buttery spread that can be served as an easy appetizer or added to dressings, sauces, soups, and pasta dishes. Our personal fave is Zucchini Quinotto with Roasted Garlic (page 145).

---

1 or more garlic bulbs

1 teaspoon olive oil per bulb

⅛ teaspoon fine sea salt per bulb

1. Preheat the oven to 400°F. Slice off the top ¼ inch of the garlic bulb(s) and remove any loose outer papery layers.

2. Place each bulb on a separate sheet of aluminum foil, drizzle with the oil, and sprinkle with salt. Wrap the foil tightly around the entire bulb.

3. Place in the center of the oven and roast until soft and golden, 40 to 50 minutes. Cool enough to handle, then squeeze from the bottom to pop each clove out of its paper.

PICKLED BEETS WITH STAR ANISE AND CINNAMON

MAKES 2 (1-PINT) JARS

for an anti-inflammatory kick

Our favorite way to devour these pickled beets is on top of salad greens with goat cheese, Wildwood Hazelnuts (page 65), and Basic Balsamic Vinaigrette (page 169).

By now you've probably noticed that we have a serious crush on beets. We put beets in smoothies (page 28), hummus (page 73), and broth (page 111) and even use the greens in pesto (page 67). But once we tried these sweetly spiced pickled beets, we just had to sneak one more vibrant red recipe into our book. Pickled beets are a weeknight dinner savior. When you peer into your fridge and think you've got zilch to top a salad, you'll remember your jar of pickled beets and thank us.

For this recipe, we consulted with Portland's root vegetable guru, cookbook author and guiding friend Diane Morgan. This beloved recipe comes straight out of her James Beard award-winning cookbook, *Roots*. It is best made 3 days in advance to give the beets time to pickle.

---

1 pound cooked red beets (see page 29), cooled, peeled, and cut into ¼-inch-thick slices

⅓ cup thinly sliced shallots

2 cups apple cider vinegar

½ cup water

½ cup coconut sugar or firmly packed light brown sugar

1 tablespoon fine sea salt

1½-inch piece cinnamon stick, broken in half

10 whole cloves

2 star anise pods

1 teaspoon whole allspice

1. Wash two 1-pint heatproof jars with tight-fitting lids in hot, soapy water and dry thoroughly. Alternatively, run the jars through the regular cycle of your dishwasher and wash the lids by hand.

2. In a large bowl, toss together the beets and shallots. Pack the jars evenly with the beet mixture and set aside.

3. In a medium saucepan, combine the vinegar, water, sugar, salt, cinnamon, cloves, star anise, and allspice. Bring to a boil over high heat, stirring constantly until the sugar dissolves. Boil the pickling liquid for 1 minute, then remove from the heat.

4. Using a wide-mouthed funnel, ladle the hot pickling liquid into the prepared jars, covering the beet mixture completely and leaving ½-inch head space. Distribute the whole spices that sink to the bottom of the saucepan evenly between the jars, making sure each jar of beets has a piece of cinnamon, a star anise, and an equal amount of cloves and allspice. Wipe the rims clean and attach the lids.

5. Let the beets steep at room temperature until cool, then store in the refrigerator for at least 3 days to allow the flavors to permeate the beets. They will keep in the refrigerator for up to 1 month.

TURMERIC PEPITAS

MAKES 2 CUPS

for a recovery snack

Shalane craves pumpkin seeds (aka pepitas). Sounds like an odd craving outside of Halloween night, but pumpkin seeds are high in protein, omega-3 fatty acids, and minerals (including iron!), which makes them a superb recovery food.

Our Turmeric Pepitas hit all the high notes since they're sweet, salty, buttery, and lightly spiced. We spike them with our favorite inflammation-fighting powerhouse—turmeric! We snack on these seeds for an afternoon boost (they make a great alternative to nuts), and we keep a jar on hand for transferring salads from blah to ah-haa! They'll steal the spotlight on top of our Recovery Quinoa Salad (page 99) or any quinoa salad for that matter.

1 tablespoon butter

1 teaspoon turmeric

1 teaspoon curry powder

2 tablespoons honey

½ teaspoon fine sea salt

2 cups raw, shelled pepitas

1. Preheat the oven to 350°F. Line a baking sheet with parchment paper.

2. Melt the butter on medium-low in a medium skillet or sauce-pan. Add the turmeric and curry powder and cook until fragrant, stirring continuously, about 1 minute. Turn off the heat and stir in the honey and salt. Add the pepitas and stir to coat.

3. Spread the pepitas on the baking sheet and roast in the center of the oven for 10 minutes, stirring after 5 minutes. They'll look moist right out of the oven but will crisp up when they cool.

4. Cool completely in a single layer, then break apart any clusters and transfer to a glass jar.

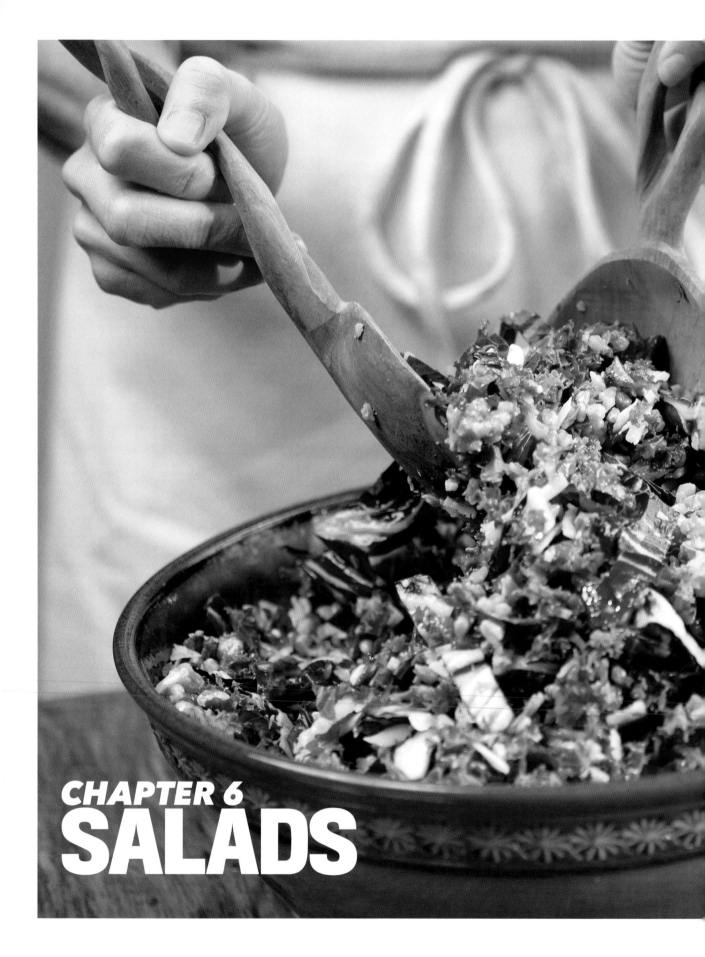

CHAPTER 6
SALADS

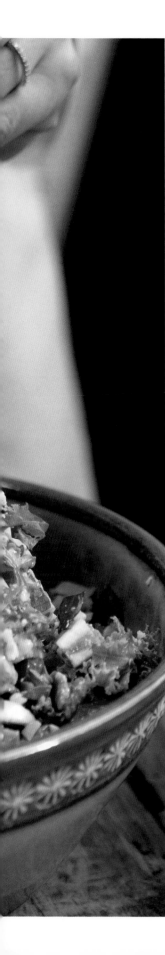

KALE-RADICCHIO SALAD WITH FARRO

SERVES 8

for bone-building nourishment

Cook times for farro vary depending on if it is whole, pearled, or semi-pearled. Quick-cooking farro lacks the nutty flavor and texture of whole farro. Our favorite is Bob's Red Mill organic farro, which is "scratched" to decrease the cook time without compromising flavor or nutrition.

As the idea for this book developed, Shalane started keeping a food journal. One of the things we realized was that she was eating countless spinach salads. While spinach is high in vitamins and minerals, in its raw state it is also high in oxalic acid, which can interfere with mineral absorption. Not good for bone health.

Enter kale salads. This was the salad Elyse brought to a summer dinner at Shalane's house the night the idea for this cookbook was born. The al dente texture of the farro combined with the lemon and garlic flavors in the dressing make this salad reminiscent of a bowl of fresh pasta. If you like, go ahead and double up on the dressing. It's chock-full of immune-boosting garlic and digestion-enhancing miso.

Elite marathoner and recipe tester Matt Llano claims to eat this salad now nearly every day. He's addicted to topping it with sliced avocado. When he can't find radicchio, he swaps in red cabbage.

1 cup farro, rinsed and drained

1 recipe Lemon Miso Dressing (page 168)

1 large bunch kale, finely chopped, stems removed

1 small head radicchio, quartered, cored, and cut crosswise into thin strips

1 cup grated Parmesan cheese

1 cup chopped toasted walnuts

1. In a large pot, place the farro with enough water to cover by a couple of inches and bring to a boil over high heat. Reduce the heat to low and simmer, covered, until the farro is tender but still chewy, about 30 minutes (see Stopwatch icon above). Drain the farro and set aside to cool.

2. To assemble the salad, toss the kale with three-quarters of the dressing in a large salad bowl. With clean hands, gently massage the kale with the dressing to soften the leaves. Add the radicchio, Parmesan, walnuts, and farro to the kale and toss again. Taste and add the remaining dressing, if needed.

3. This salad can be made in advance. It tastes even better the second day. Cover and refrigerate leftovers for up to 5 days.

STRAWBERRY-ARUGULA KAMUT SALAD

SERVES 5

for a revitalizing summer dinner

For easy grain salads all summer long, we highly recommend cooking a big batch of Kamut berries and freezing them in individually portioned freezer bags. Simply take a bag of grains out of the freezer and thaw on the counter an hour prior to tossing in a salad.

This hearty and refreshing salad is a cinch to toss together for a light, yet completely satisfying, summer dinner or a memorable side dish. Bring this dish to an alfresco BBQ and you'll have everyone begging for the recipe.

Elyse added Kamut berries to her grains repertoire after meeting Maria Speck, who was on tour for her second cookbook, *Simply Ancient Grains*. Kamut, an ancient wheat variety, is revered for its rich nutty flavor, addictively chewy texture, and energy-giving nutrition. It's higher in protein, selenium, amino acids, and vitamin E than most modern wheat and contains essential minerals such as magnesium and zinc.

If you can't find Kamut berries or other wheat berries, swap in farro (opposite page), which cooks faster and doesn't need to be soaked overnight.

---

1 cup Kamut berries, soaked overnight and drained, or about 2½ cups cooked

1 teaspoon fine sea salt

5 cups loosely packed arugula

2 cups sliced strawberries

1 recipe Basic Balsamic Vinaigrette (page 169)

½ cup crumbled ricotta salata or feta cheese

½ cup chopped toasted hazelnuts (or Wildwood Hazelnuts, page 65)

1. Bring 4 cups of water to a boil in a large heavy saucepan. Add the Kamut and salt and simmer, covered, until soft with a slight chew, 50 to 60 minutes. Use a fine-mesh sieve to drain thoroughly.

2. Transfer the Kamut to a large salad bowl and spread out to cool.

3. Once cool, combine with the arugula and strawberries. Just before serving, toss with three-fourths of the dressing, taste, and add more dressing, if needed. Top with the cheese and nuts.

OREGON SUMMER SALAD WITH GRILLED SALMON

SERVES 2

for endless summer nights

When we visit the Portland Farmers Market in the summertime, here's what you'll find in our basket: wild salmon, asparagus, berries, hazelnuts, artisan goat cheese, arugula, farm-fresh eggs, and a loaf of bread from a local bakery. Years ago, Elyse decided to combine all these seasonal favorites into one salad (minus the eggs), and our beloved Oregon Summer Salad was born.

When the evenings are just too perfect to be spent inside cooking, we find ourselves making this quick and easy salad on a near weekly basis. We like to toss the salmon on the grill, but it can also be cooked in minutes under the broiler. Or if you want to get dinner on the table pronto, buy hot-smoked (already cooked) salmon—and the asparagus can be sliced thin and left raw, or substitute any assortment of leftover grilled veggies.

1 tablespoon olive oil

¾ pound wild salmon or arctic char, cut into 2 fillets

½ pound asparagus, trimmed

½ teaspoon coarse sea salt

¼ teaspoon freshly ground black pepper

3 cups loosely packed arugula or other salad greens

½ cup blueberries

½ cup chopped toasted hazelnuts (or Wildwood Hazelnuts, page 65)

½ cup crumbled goat cheese or feta cheese

1 recipe Basic Balsamic Vinaigrette (page 169)

1. Preheat the grill to medium-high or preheat the broiler with an oven rack set on the upper shelf.

2. Drizzle the oil over the salmon and asparagus and sprinkle with the salt and pepper. Grill the salmon until opaque, 2 to 3 minutes per side, depending on the thickness of the fillet. At the same time, grill the asparagus, rotating frequently, until lightly charred, 3 to 4 minutes. Remove to a clean plate. Alternatively, place the salmon and asparagus on a baking sheet lined with foil. Cook under the broiler until the salmon is opaque, 6 to 10 minutes (depending on the thickness of the fillet), and the asparagus is lightly charred, 3 to 4 minutes (rotating frequently). If the asparagus are done, but the salmon needs more time, remove the asparagus to a cutting board and return the salmon to the oven.

3. Pile 2 large salad bowls with the arugula or salad greens. Top with the blueberries, hazelnuts, and cheese.

4. Slice the asparagus into 2-inch pieces. Top each salad with a salmon fillet and the asparagus and drizzle with the dressing. Serve with a slice of crusty bread, if desired.

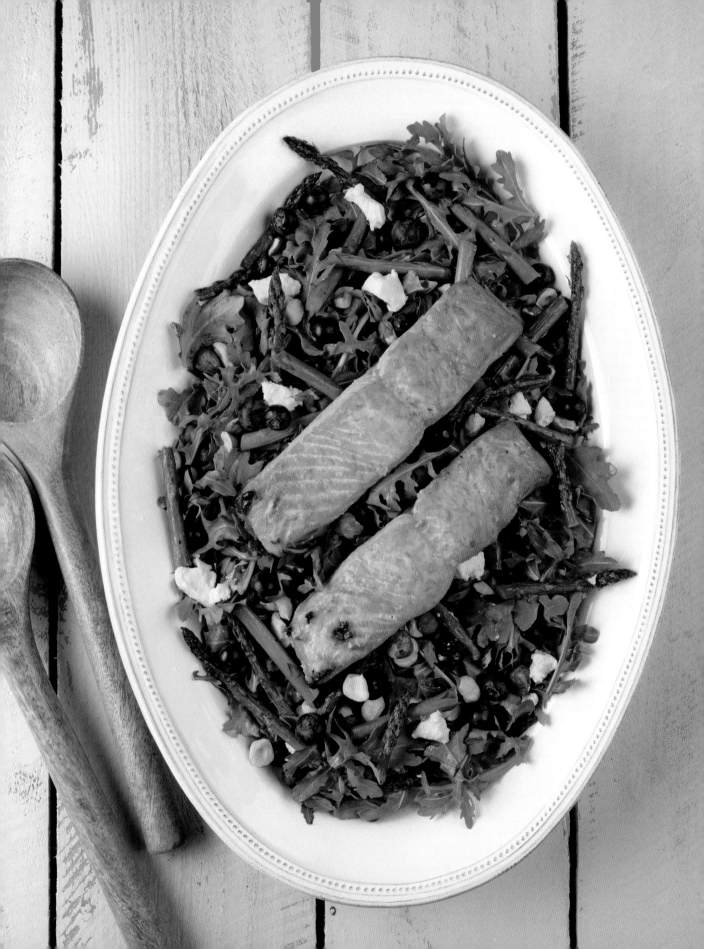

ROOT LOVERS' WINTER SALAD

SERVES 4

for a colorful antioxidant boost

Colorful salads need not be reserved for the summer months. Come winter, not a week goes by that we aren't roasting a tray full of vibrant root vegetables. Roasted roots can be served as a simple side dish, but we like them best tossed with spicy arugula and drizzled with a creamy tangy dressing to highlight their earthy sweetness.

Our favorite combination is beets, carrots, parsnips, and rutabaga, but feel free to mix it up to your liking. To ensure even cooking, chop all roots roughly the same size.

We promise moos, oinks, clucks, and quacks won't be missed when you serve this salad as a vegetarian main dish.

---

2 pounds root vegetables (carrots, beets, parsnips, rutabaga, turnips, potatoes), peeled and cut into 1-inch pieces (about 6 cups)

2 tablespoons extra-virgin olive oil

1 teaspoon ground cumin

½ teaspoon fine sea salt

¼ teaspoon ground red pepper

1 can (15 ounces) chickpeas, drained, rinsed, and patted dry, or 1½ cups cooked chickpeas

1 red onion, halved, cut into wedges

5 cups arugula or other hearty salad greens

1 recipe Creamy Apple Cider Vinaigrette (page 173)

1. Preheat the oven to 425°F. Line a rimmed baking sheet with parchment paper.

2. In a large mixing bowl, combine the root vegetables and oil. Add the cumin, salt, and red pepper and stir until evenly coated.

3. Spread the vegetables out on the baking sheet and roast in the center of the oven for 30 to 45 minutes, stirring every 15 minutes. After 15 minutes, toss the chickpeas and onions with the veggies and return to the oven, until the roots are soft when pierced with a fork and evenly browned.

4. Transfer the roasted veggies to a large salad bowl, toss with the arugula, and serve immediately with the dressing on the side for drizzling over top.

NOSTRANA'S PASTA SALAD

SERVES 8

for a mayo-free crowd pleaser

Forget the American version of pasta salad consisting of over-cooked spiral noodles drowning in mayo with chunks of processed ham and a sliver of something resembling a vegetable. For this recipe, we consulted with our favorite Italian cuisine connoisseur, Chef Cathy Whims. With six James Beard Award nominations under her belt and 10 years overseeing the incredible kitchen at Nostrana, in Portland, Oregon, Chef Cathy knows how to work magical simplicity into classic Italian fare. And like us, she relocated to Portland from Chapel Hill, North Carolina.

This recipe is crazy simple. The key is to seek out the highest-quality ingredients you can get. Top-shelf olive oil is worth its weight in gold, and dried pasta made from semolina or durum wheat is preferable.

The recipe below makes enough pasta salad to feed a party of eight. It can be easily cut in half, if desired.

4 red bell peppers, seeded and cut into 1-inch pieces

2 eggplants, cut into ½-inch cubes

2 fennel bulbs, quartered, cored, and cut into 1-inch pieces

½ cup high-quality extra-virgin olive oil

1¾ teaspoons coarse sea salt

1 pound dried penne, farfalle, or fusilli

1 cup grated Parmesan cheese

½ cup pitted, chopped kalamata olives

1 cup chopped fresh parsley and/or fresh basil

¼ cup lemon juice

½ teaspoon freshly ground black pepper

1. Preheat the oven to 425°F.

2. In an extra-large mixing bowl, toss the bell peppers, eggplants, and fennel with ¼ cup of the oil and 1 teaspoon of the salt. Spread out on 2 baking sheets and roast in the center and lower racks of the oven until lightly charred, 30 to 40 minutes, stirring every 15 minutes.

3. Cook the pasta in heavily salted boiling water according to package directions until al dente (which is preferred). Drain and rinse under cold water. Transfer to an extra-large salad bowl and toss immediately with the remaining ¼ cup oil.

4. Add the roasted vegetables, Parmesan, olives, parsley or basil, lemon juice, black pepper, and the remaining ¾ teaspoon salt to the salad bowl and toss well. Taste and add more salt, if needed.

5. Serve warm or at room temperature.

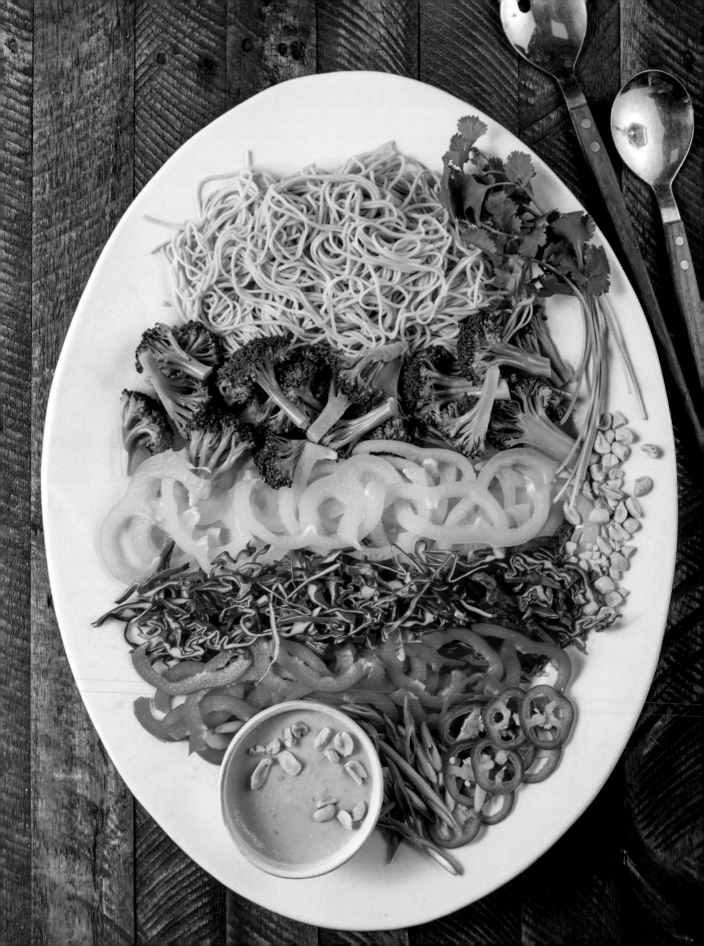

SOBA NOODLE SALAD WITH RUNNER'S HIGH PEANUT SAUCE

SERVES 4

for inspired Sunday dinners

1 tablespoon fine sea salt

1 head broccoli, cut into bite-size florets

¼ small purple or white cabbage

1 package (8 to 9.5 ounces) soba noodles (buckwheat noodles)

1 tablespoon toasted sesame oil

1 tablespoon soy sauce (preferably shoyu or tamari)

1 red or yellow bell pepper, quartered and seeded

½ cup loosely packed chopped cilantro leaves

4 or 5 scallions, roots trimmed, white and green parts sliced

1 jalapeño chile pepper, stem removed, sliced thin (wear plastic gloves when handling) or small bowl of kimchi (optional, if you like spice)

½ cup chopped roasted peanuts

1½ cups Runner's High Peanut Sauce (page 175)

The peanut sauce can be made up to 3 days in advance. Or better yet, make a double batch of the sauce and freeze what you don't use for future Soba Sundays.

This recipe came to be when Shalane's mom, Cheryl Treworgy, a former marathon world record holder (yes, Shalane has good genes!), told us she was drizzling our addicting Runner's High Peanut Sauce (page 175) on salads. At that moment, we knew we needed to create a salad worthy of our luscious sauce.

Kids and kids-at-heart will love this deconstructed Soba Noodle Salad, which allows everyone sitting around the table to build their own beautiful bowl of goodness. Start a Soba Sunday Tradition and serve up a different array of colorful veggies every week. Try mixing in grated carrots, jicama, bean sprouts, edamame, or leftover grilled chicken, steak, shrimp, or tempeh.

1. Bring a large pot of water to a rolling boil over high heat and add the salt. Place the broccoli and cabbage in the water for 2 minutes. Remove from the water and immediately transfer to a large bowl of ice water to stop the cooking (and keep the veggies crisp). Once the vegetables are chilled, remove them from the water and set aside.

2. Bring the same pot of water back up to a rolling boil and cook the noodles according to the package directions. Drain, run under cold water, drain again thoroughly, and transfer to a large salad bowl. Toss the noodles with the sesame oil and soy sauce.

3. Thinly slice the cabbage and bell pepper (use a mandoline if you have one). Arrange the broccoli, cabbage, bell pepper, cilantro, scallions, and chile pepper or kimchi (if using) on a large platter alongside the noodles. Place the peanuts in a small bowl.

4. Warm the peanut sauce in a small saucepan over low heat. Transfer to a medium bowl.

5. Place the platter in the center of the table and allow everyone to create their own soba noodle salads. Top with a generous serving of the peanut sauce.

GREEN APPLE-FENNEL SALAD WITH HAZELNUTS

SERVES 4

for boosting digestion

Even when the weather starts to turn cold, refreshing salads remain a must in every athlete's diet. Filling your plate with raw vegetables ensures you're getting an adequate dose of enzymes to keep your digestive and immune systems working at their best. And a salad need not be dull. This sophisticated salad was inspired by all things good about fall in our home state of Oregon.

1 large fennel bulb, top sliced off, quartered, fronds minced

1 large Granny Smith apple, quartered and cored

½ cup crumbled ricotta salata or feta cheese

½ cup chopped toasted hazelnuts or walnuts

½ cup pitted, chopped dates (optional)

1 recipe Apple Cider Vinaigrette (page 173)

Freshly ground black pepper

1. Slice out the hard inner core at the bottom of the fennel quarters. Thinly slice the fennel and apple and place in a large salad bowl. Add the fennel fronds, cheese, nuts, and dates (if using).

2. Pour three-fourths of the dressing over the salad and toss. Taste and add more dressing, if needed. Grind fresh pepper over top. Serve with a crusty baguette, if desired.

Got hungry dinner guests? Serve this with our Bacon-Wrapped Stuffed Chicken (page 129).

Slicing the apple and fennel with a mandoline set at ⅛ inch or a high-quality chef's knife will save you time and help you achieve crunchy perfection. The first time Shalane used a mandoline, she cut herself, so please be careful and use the safety guard.

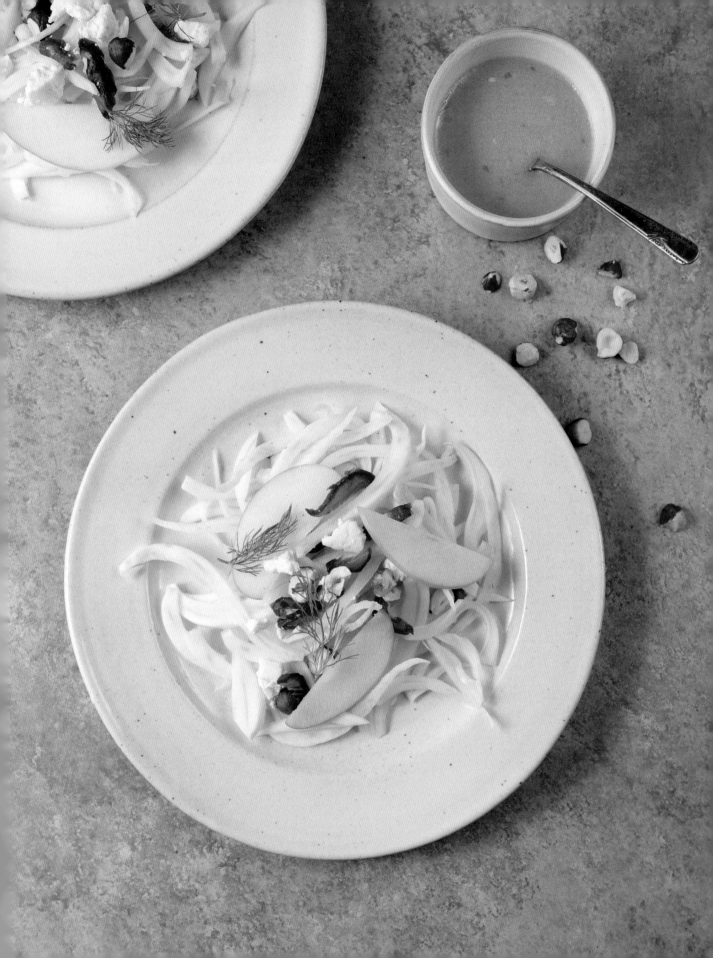

WILD WEST RICE SALAD

SERVES 4

for a vegan recovery meal

 To save time, use a food processor or high-speed blender to pulse the veggies until finely chopped.

Go wild. Experiment with adding your own combination of favorite seasonal veggies. Think tomatoes and bell peppers in the summer and roasted root vegetables in the winter.

Call us crazy, but sometimes we get tired of quinoa salads. But we love grain salads because they're simple enough to make on a weekly basis and hearty enough to stand alone as a complete meal (great for lunch all week long). And so we got to cookin' other grains for salads, including wild rice (here), farro (page 80), and Kamut berries (page 81).

For vegetarians and vegans alike, getting all nine essential amino acids (the building blocks of protein) into your diet can be a challenge. While meat has all nine naturally, grains and beans are not a complete protein. Fear not. Combine them and—bada-bing!— they're complete. That's why we've tossed vibrant edamame into this colorful whole grain salad.

Fill up and you'll be ready to take on your meat-loving competition!

½ teaspoon fine sea salt, plus more to taste

1 cup wild rice, rinsed

Double batch of Creamy Apple Cider Vinaigrette (page 173)

6 radishes, diced

3 cups loosely packed, finely chopped kale, stems removed

3 carrots, grated

6 scallions, white and green parts, thinly sliced

1 cup frozen shelled edamame, cooked according to package directions

Freshly ground black pepper

1. Bring 4 cups water and the salt to a boil in a large saucepan. Add the rice, reduce the heat, cover, and simmer until the rice grains burst open and are soft but chewy, 35 to 40 minutes.

2. Drain the rice, transfer to a large salad bowl, and immediately toss with half the dressing.

3. Allow the rice to cool, then add the radishes, kale, carrots, scallions, and edamame and toss until combined.

4. Add more dressing and salt and pepper to taste.

5. Let the salad marinate in the fridge for at least 30 minutes prior to serving.

TIP

When cooking rice for salads, it's best to slightly undercook the grain to maintain a satisfying chewy, al dente texture that can hold up to the dressing.

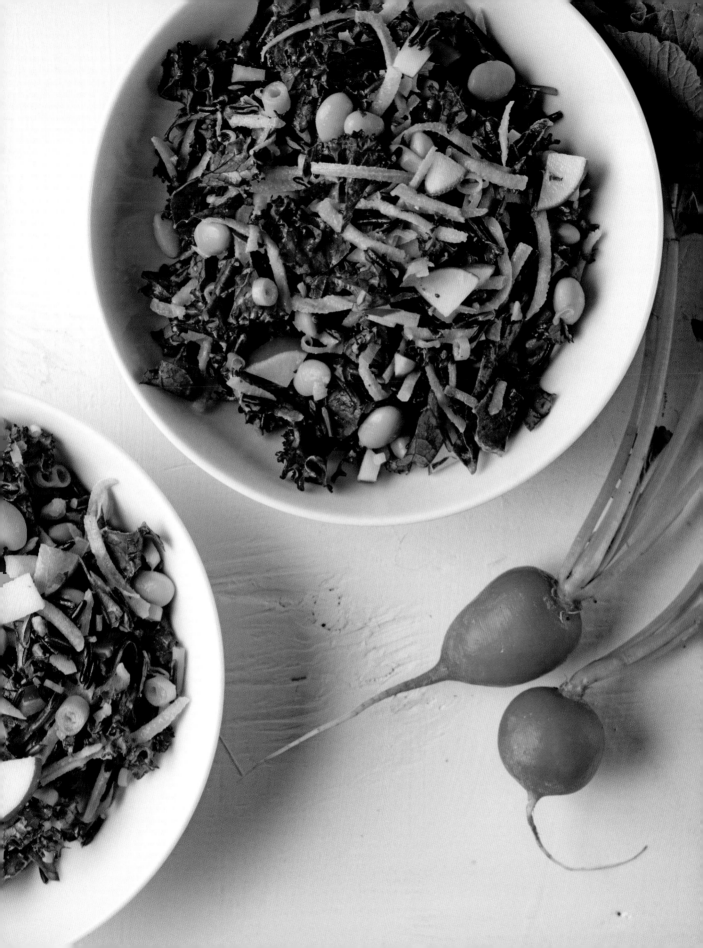

CAROLINA TARRAGON CHICKEN SALAD

SERVES 6

for creamy richness without mayo

1½ pounds boneless, skinless chicken breasts and thighs (or about 3½ cups shredded cooked chicken)

1 teaspoon extra-virgin olive oil

½ teaspoon fine sea salt, plus more to taste

¼ teaspoon freshly ground black pepper, plus more to taste

½ cup mashed ripe avocado (about 1 avocado)

¼ cup plain whole milk yogurt

¼ cup finely chopped fresh tarragon leaves

1 tablespoon finely chopped shallot

2 tablespoons lemon juice

1 large Granny Smith apple, chopped

3 ribs celery, thinly sliced

½ cup chopped toasted walnuts

4 cups loosely packed arugula or other salad greens

This recipe is a throwback to our Carolina days. In college, at UNC, we lived together in a shabby and not-at-all-chic duplex. Lucky for us there was a fabulous little deli, called Foster's Market, just across the street. When hunger struck, and the fridge was intimidatingly overstuffed with long-expired and inedible leftovers, we would bolt across the street and fill up on our favorite dish, Tarragon Chicken Salad.

Since store-bought mayo (even the organic brands) is full of cheap hydrogenated oils, sugar, and preservatives, our cookbook assistant, Natalie Bickford, suggested testing a version with yogurt. Combining the yogurt with mashed avocado lent the creamy richness we craved, without the unhealthy additives.

1. Preheat the oven to 400°F.

2. Rub the chicken with the oil, generously sprinkle with salt and pepper, and roast on a baking sheet in the center of the oven until a thermometer inserted in the thickest portion registers 165°F and the juices run clear, 15 minutes. Allow the chicken to cool for 10 minutes, then transfer to a cutting board and use two forks to shred it. Place uncovered in the fridge to cool completely.

3. In a large salad bowl, whisk together the avocado, yogurt, tarragon, shallot, lemon juice, ½ teaspoon salt, and ¼ teaspoon pepper. Add the chicken, apple, celery, and walnuts and stir to combine. Taste and add additional salt and pepper, if needed.

4. Chill in the fridge until ready to serve. Place on top of a bed of arugula or other salad greens. Serve with a hunk of crusty baguette, if desired.

5. Store in an airtight container in the fridge for up to 3 days.

Celebrate chicken thighs. Not only is dark meat richer in flavor, it's also richer in muscle-building nutrients. It will leave you feeling satisfied longer and is less expensive.

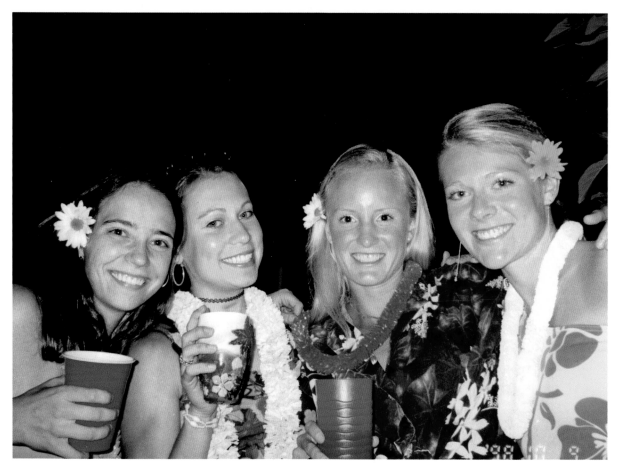

Shalane and Elyse celebrating after a cross-country race in 2003 with fellow UNC roommates, Alice Kehaya and Monica Mannino.

TIP
Tarragon has a lovely licorice aroma that gives
this salad a unique twist, but if you can't find tarragon,
substitute in fresh basil.

OMEGA SARDINE SALAD

SERVES 2

for training like an Olympian

Still not willing to forgo your tuna salad? Hear us out. Sardines are sustainable, free from contaminants like mercury, and far healthier than their big fish counterpart.

You've probably heard that sardines are an amazing power food but never thought they'd be something you'd actually want to eat. Now you will. This omega-3-loaded variation on the traditional tuna salad makes a regular appearance in our lunch repertoire. It's made with ingredients that are easy to keep stocked, so you have no excuse not to take the time to make this energizing lunch.

From the sardines, eggs, yogurt, and walnuts, you'll get a serious dose of essential fatty acids, important for everything from fighting inflammation to boosting your mood. Plus, did you know that eggs have all nine essential amino acids, making them a complete protein and the perfect recovery food?

The creamy tanginess from the yogurt and Dijon mustard offsets any fishiness. The celery and walnuts add crunch. We like to serve this salad piled on top of thick slices of whole grain toast with a simple green salad.

This salad was Amy Cragg's go-to recovery lunch in her training leading up to winning the 2016 Olympic Marathon Trials.

---

2 hard-boiled eggs, peeled (see Tip)

2 ribs celery, chopped

¼ cup minced fresh parsley

¼ cup plain whole milk Greek yogurt

2 teaspoons Dijon mustard

1 can (4.25 ounces) sardines in olive oil, drained

¼ cup toasted chopped walnuts

¼ cup pitted, chopped kalamata olives

Fine sea salt

Freshly ground black pepper

In a medium bowl, smash the eggs with the back of a fork to break them up. Add the celery, parsley, yogurt, and mustard and stir to combine. Add the sardines, walnuts, and olives and stir to break up the sardines into bite-size pieces. Season to taste with salt and ground pepper.

TIP

To make perfect hard-boiled eggs, place the eggs in a medium saucepan with enough water to fully submerge. Bring to a rolling boil, cover, turn off the heat, remove from the burner, and let stand for 10 minutes. Drain and transfer to a bowl of cold water. Once cool, store in the fridge or peel if using right away.

PESTO POTATO SALAD

SERVES 5

for a mayo-free take on a classic

For dinner parties, we recommend doubling the recipe. You'll want leftovers. This salad will keep for up to 5 days.

We snuck this recipe into our cookbook as a late addition by special request. Elyse served this refreshing interpretation of potato salad at a family picnic and was asked, "Is this recipe in the book? It should be!" And so it came to be.

Gloppy mayo-loaded potato salad, move aside. This Pesto Potato Salad will steal the limelight at your next backyard BBQ. Not only is it better for you, it also won't spoil as quickly since it's mayo-free.

If you listened to us and made a double batch of our Arugula Cashew Pesto (page 67), then after cooking the potatoes, you'll be able to pull this dish together faster than Shalane can run a mile. That means in under 4 minutes and 23 seconds!

---

2 pounds red potatoes, cut into 1-inch pieces

1 tablespoon + ½ teaspoon fine sea salt

1 cup Arugula Cashew Pesto (page 67)

1 tablespoon lemon juice

¼ teaspoon freshly ground black pepper

1. In a large saucepan, place the potatoes, 1 tablespoon salt, and enough water to cover by a couple of inches. Bring to a boil over high heat, then reduce the heat to low and simmer, uncovered, until the potatoes are tender but not mushy when pierced with a fork, 10 to 15 minutes.

2. Drain the potatoes and place in a large salad bowl. Allow them to cool for 5 minutes. While still warm, gently toss with the pesto, lemon juice, pepper, and ½ teaspoon salt until combined. Taste and add additional salt and pepper, if needed. Serve warm or at room temperature.

3. If making in advance, store covered in the fridge and take out 1 hour prior to serving.

MOROCCAN LENTIL SALAD WITH CAULIFLOWER COUSCOUS

SERVES 6

for inflammation-fighting happiness

1 cup dried green lentils, sorted and rinsed

½ teaspoon fine sea salt

3 medium carrots, peeled and grated (or pulsed in a food processor)

2 cups loosely packed, chopped kale, stems removed

½ cup chopped toasted pistachios or almonds

½ cup chopped dried Turkish apricots

¼ cup pitted, chopped kalamata olives

1 tablespoon ras el hanout (Moroccan spice blend)

5 cups Cauliflower Couscous (page 156) or 1 cup uncooked couscous (prepare according to package directions)

Double recipe Maple-Dijon Apple Cider Vinaigrette (page 173)

This hearty salad takes longer to prep than a monotonous spinach salad but is well worth the effort—one bowlful is a complete meal in itself. It stores fabulously, making it the perfect dish to serve on a Sunday night with hopes of having enough leftovers for lunch.

For those who are sensitive to grains or who want to lighten the load on their digestive systems, we highly recommend making the "couscous" out of cauliflower. When we served it this way, both our husbands failed to notice the couscous was missing. (Don't tell!)

Ras el hanout is an incredible Moroccan spice blend that Elyse fell hard for while taking culinary classes in Marrakesh. It's loaded with sweet inflammation-fighting spices. You can find it in most high-quality grocery stores, or you can make your own simplified blend (see Tip below).

1. Place the lentils in a medium pot, add the salt, and cover with 2 inches of water. Bring to a boil over high heat, then reduce the heat to low, cover, and simmer until tender but not mushy, 25 to 30 minutes. Drain and set aside to cool.

2. Place the carrots, kale, nuts, apricots, olives, and ras el hanout in a large salad bowl. Add the couscous and lentils and toss until evenly combined. Add two-thirds of the dressing, toss, and taste. Add more dressing to taste, if needed.

3. Cover the salad and place in the fridge to chill for at least 30 minutes or until ready to serve.

TIP

Make your own simple Moroccan spice blend. Substitute the tablespoon of ras el hanout with 1 teaspoon ground cumin, 1 teaspoon turmeric, 1 teaspoon ground cinnamon, and ¼ teaspoon freshly ground black pepper.

Cook the lentils with a 1-inch piece of kombu to add minerals and make them more digestible.

To save time, skip chopping each ingredient by hand and instead put your food processor or high-speed blender to work for you. Each ingredient can be individually pulsed until chopped.

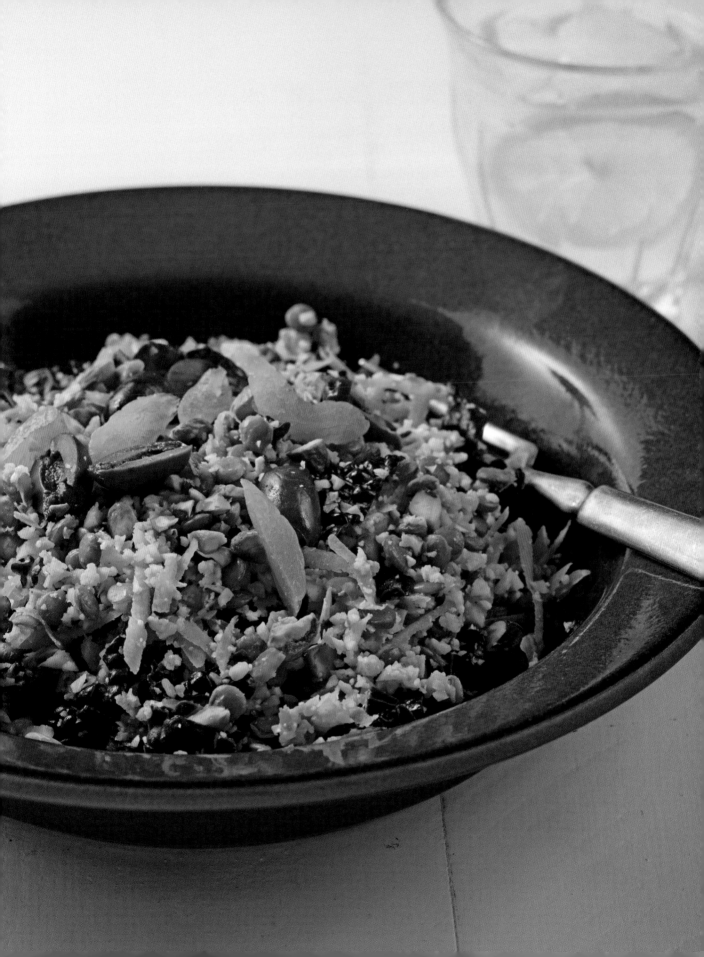

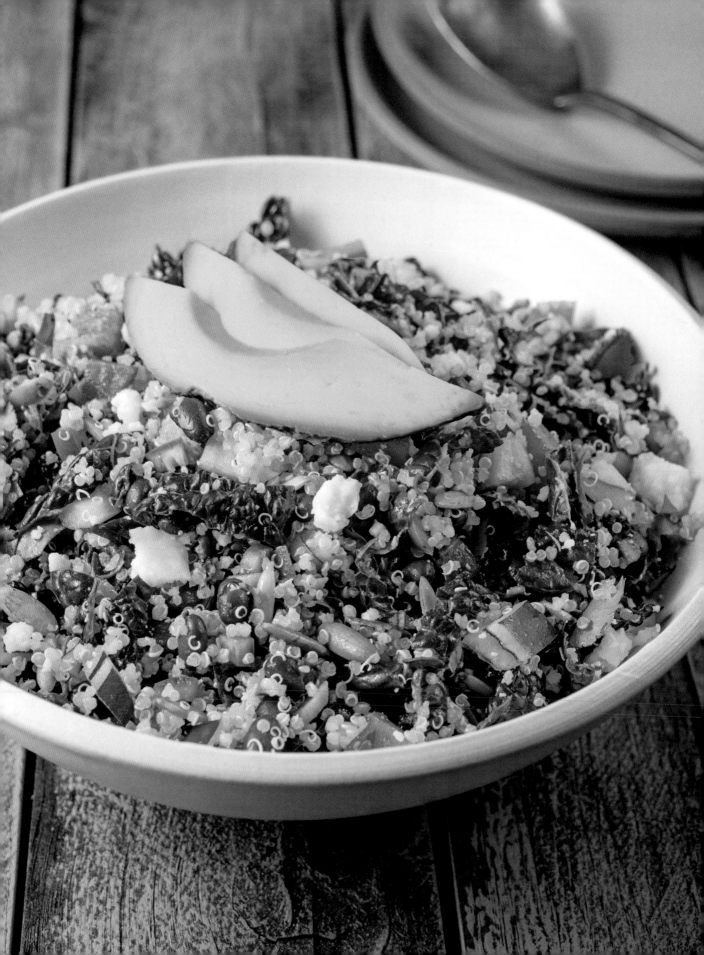

RECOVERY QUINOA SALAD

SERVES 6

for a salad that cures

1 cup quinoa, rinsed using a fine-mesh strainer

¾ teaspoon fine sea salt

3 cups loosely packed, finely chopped kale, stems removed

1 red bell pepper, seeded and chopped

1 jalapeño chile pepper, finely chopped (include the seeds if you like spice), wear plastic gloves when handling

½ small red onion, chopped

½ cup chopped cilantro leaves

1 can (15 ounces) black beans, drained and rinsed, or 1½ cups cooked black beans

⅓ cup lime juice (3 or 4 limes)

⅓ cup extra-virgin olive oil

1 avocado, sliced

½ cup toasted pumpkin seeds (see Tip on page 62) or Turmeric Pepitas (page 77)

½ cup grated Cotija, crumbled feta cheese, or chopped olives

For this recipe, we went to the drawing boards—the social media boards, that is, and asked you to share your favorite quinoa salad pairings. The resounding winner was a Mexican-themed quinoa salad complete with black beans, avocado, cilantro, and lime. We didn't think you would mind, but we also snuck in a few more veggies and topped the salad with our Turmeric Pepitas (page 77).

We found this salad so refreshing and revitalizing that we now call it our Recovery Salad. For vegans and vegetarians (and meat lovers), quinoa is fantastic after a hard workout since it's the only plant food containing all nine essential amino acids—essential for repairing those sore muscles.

1. In a medium saucepan over high heat, bring to a boil the quinoa, 1½ cups water, and ½ teaspoon of the salt. Reduce the heat to low and simmer, covered, until the quinoa is tender and all the water has been absorbed, 15 to 20 minutes. Transfer to a large salad bowl, fluff with a fork, and set aside to cool.

2. Once cool, add the kale, red bell pepper, chile pepper, onion, cilantro, black beans, lime juice, oil, and the remaining ¼ teaspoon salt to the quinoa and toss to combine. Taste and add additional salt, if needed. Chill in the fridge until ready to serve.

3. Just before serving, top with the avocado slices, pumpkin seeds or Turmeric Pepitas, and the cheese or olives.

TIP

If you don't like the bite or aftertaste of raw onion, soak the chopped onion in a small bowl of cold water for 10 minutes. Then drain and add to the salad.

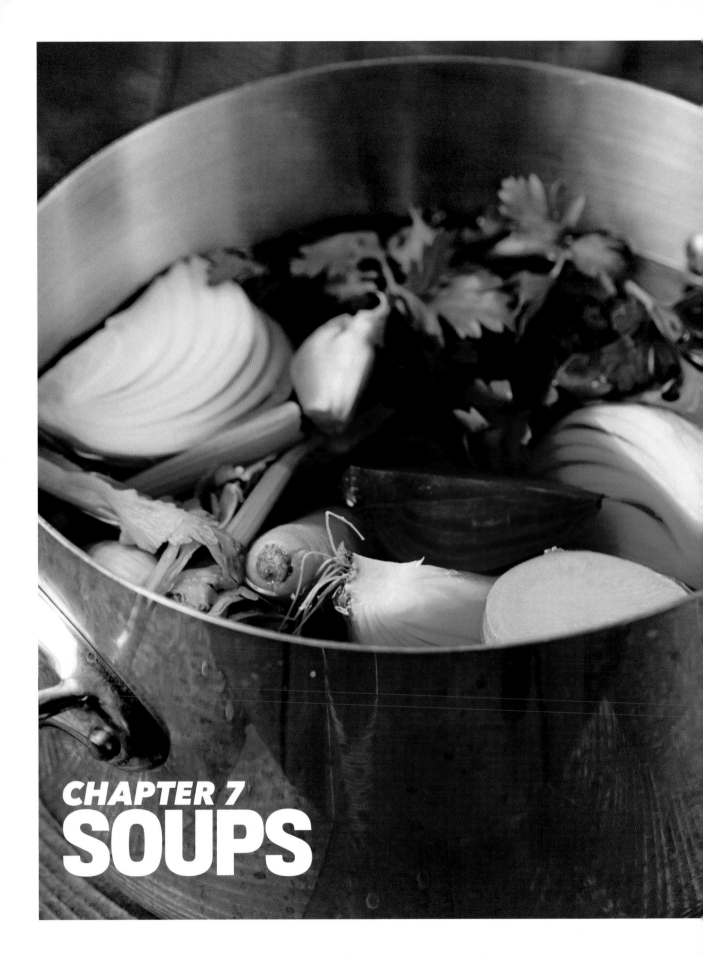

CHAPTER 7
SOUPS

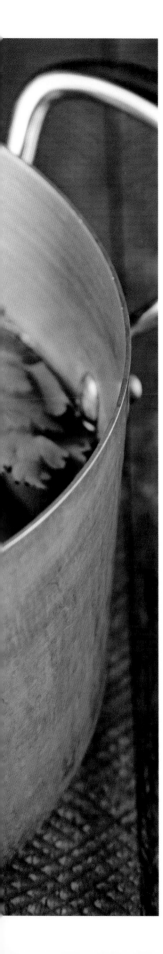

BROCCOLI CHÈVRE SOUP

SERVES 4

for nourished comfort

Our love affair with Switzerland and Swiss-inspired cuisine began in our college days. The summer after our junior year, we and our fellow track teammate and roommate, Alice Kehaya, took a break from running to backpack through Europe. While traveling through Switzerland, we happily lived off bread and cheese and fell hard for fresh goat's cheese, also called chèvre.

As a nod to our unforgettable backpack adventure, Elyse was inspired to makeover the classic American broccoli cheddar soup with fresh chèvre. Not only is goat's cheese easier to digest for those who are sensitive to dairy, it's also higher in protein, calcium, and potassium than its mooing counterpart. Best of all, it lends a tart, tangy, earthy flavor that turns this nourishing vegetable soup into a showstopper.

2 tablespoons unsalted butter

1 yellow onion, chopped

2 carrots, peeled and chopped

1 teaspoon fine sea salt (leave out if broth is not low-sodium)

3 cloves garlic, roughly chopped

4 cups low-sodium vegetable broth or Long Run Mineral Broth (page 111)

1 large head broccoli, cut into florets

1 bay leaf

½ teaspoon freshly ground black pepper

2 tablespoons tahini (learn more about tahini on page 204)

4 ounces soft plain chèvre (goat's cheese)

1. In a large pot over medium-high heat, melt the butter. Add the onion, carrots, and salt and cook, stirring occasionally, until the onions soften but do not brown, about 5 minutes. Add the garlic and stir continuously for 1 minute longer.

2. Add the broth, broccoli, bay leaf, and pepper to the pot. Bring to a boil, then reduce the heat to low. Simmer, covered, until the broccoli and carrots are tender, 15 to 20 minutes.

3. Remove the bay leaf and turn off the heat. If you have an immersion (stick) blender, use it to blend the soup until smooth right in the pot. Alternatively, allow the soup to cool slightly, then transfer it to a blender and process until smooth. Please note: Adding hot items to a blender causes the pressure to expand and can blow off the lid, so hold it firmly in place and blend on low. Add in the tahini and chèvre and blend again until combined.

4. Taste and season with additional salt and pepper if needed. Keep warm on the stovetop until ready to serve. If the soup is too thick, thin with a little broth or water.

5. Ladle the soup into warmed bowls and top with crostini (page 68).

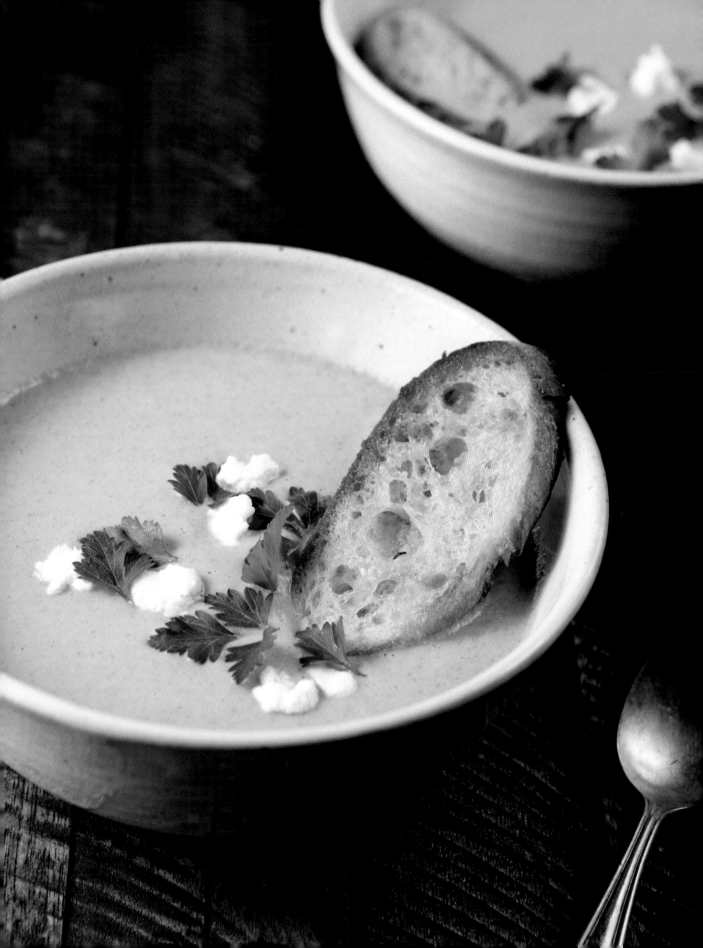

CURRY LENTIL SOUP WITH CHARRED CAULIFLOWER

SERVES 4

for rejuvenation after a winter run

1 tablespoon extra-virgin olive oil

3 carrots, chopped

1 large yellow onion, chopped

1 teaspoon fine sea salt (leave out if broth is not low-sodium)

2 cloves garlic, minced

⅛ to ¼ teaspoon red pepper flakes (optional, if you like spice)

4 cups low-sodium vegetable broth or Long Run Mineral Broth (page 111)

1 cup unsweetened full-fat coconut milk

1 cup green lentils, sorted and rinsed

2 tablespoons curry powder

3-inch-strip kombu (seaweed, page 16), optional

3 cups loosely packed, roughly chopped kale, stems removed

1 tablespoon fresh lime juice

1 recipe Charred Cauliflower (page 157), optional

Glance through the recipes in this book and you'll notice that we have a serious obsession with coconut. We put coconut water in our smoothies for an added electrolyte boost, bake with coconut oil for its buttery richness, add shredded coconut to our granola to pack in the power, and pour coconut milk into everything from soups and stews to ice cream.

Our love affair with coconut began long before we discovered its behind-the-scenes superpowers. But its benefits are unbeatable—the medium chain fatty acid in coconut is a highly usable energy source. It enhances our ability to absorb nutrients, stimulates metabolism, and boosts immunity.

This rich, fragrant, veggie-loaded soup will warm the soul and rejuvenate the body after a winter run. Forgo soggy croutons and top each bowlful with charred cauliflower for an impressive finish.

1. Heat the oil in a large pot over medium heat. Add the carrots, onion, and salt and cook, stirring occasionally, until softened but not brown, about 5 minutes. Add the garlic and pepper flakes (if using) and cook, stirring continuously, for 1 minute, being careful not to let the garlic brown.

2. Add the broth, coconut milk, lentils, curry powder, and kombu (if using). Bring to a boil, then reduce the heat and simmer covered, stirring occasionally, until the lentils are soft, 25 minutes.

3. Remove the kombu and discard. Stir in the kale and simmer for 5 minutes. Turn off the heat and stir in the lime juice. Taste and season with additional salt and pepper flakes if needed. If too thick, add ½ cup water or more until the desired consistency is reached. Serve topped with Charred Cauliflower (if desired).

FARTLEK CHILI

SERVES 6

for slowing down to speed up

2 tablespoons extra-virgin olive oil

3 carrots, peeled and finely chopped

1 large red onion, finely chopped

1½ teaspoons fine sea salt (cut in half if your broth is not low-sodium)

2 green bell peppers, seeded and chopped

1 pound ground beef (we use 85% lean grass-fed beef since the fat adds flavor; ground turkey or crumbled tempeh can also be used)

3 cloves garlic, roughly minced

2 tablespoons chili powder

2 teaspoons ground cumin

2 teaspoons ground cinnamon

¼ teaspoon ground red pepper (optional, if you like spice)

2 cups Classic Chicken Bone Broth (page 113) or store-bought low-sodium chicken or veggie broth

2 cans (14.5 ounces each) no-salt-added diced tomatoes

2 cans (15 ounces each) black, pinto, or kidney beans, drained and rinsed, or 3 cups cooked beans

Optional toppings: sour cream, grated cheese, sliced scallions, and/or Avocado Cream (page 178)

Our fellow running friends will get the joke in the naming of our chili. Google *fartlek* and you'll learn we named our chili after a type of training guaranteed to make you stronger—and not after the digestive powers that a bowl loaded with beans might prompt.

For the latter, don't come complaining to us! Our deeply spiced, cinnamon-kissed chili beckons you to come back for seconds (yes, we put cinnamon in our chili!). Elyse once won a chili cook-off thanks to her sister Jessa's genius idea to add a smidge of this sweet spice to complement the fiery heat of cayenne.

For a vegan-friendly chili, swap in crumbled tempeh for the ground beef and vegetable broth for the chicken broth, and your meat-loving friends likely won't even notice the switch-a-roo. For a mild chili, leave out the cayenne.

1. Heat the oil in a large heavy-bottomed pot over medium-high heat. Add the carrots, onion, and salt and cook, stirring occasionally, until soft but not brown, about 5 minutes.

2. Add the bell peppers, beef (or turkey or tempeh), garlic, chili powder, cumin, cinnamon, and red pepper (if using). Continuously stir, breaking up the meat into bite-size pieces, until the meat is browned, about 5 minutes.

3. Add the broth, tomatoes, and beans and bring to a simmer. Turn the heat to low, cover, and simmer for at least 30 minutes or, preferably, 1 hour.

4. Taste and add more salt (and red pepper), if needed. If too thick, thin with a little broth.

5. Serve bowls steaming-hot topped with any combination of sour cream, cheese, and scallions (if desired). Or better yet, serve topped with a spoonful of Avocado Cream (if desired).

 To make in a slow cooker: Follow steps 1 and 2, then add the cooked veggies and meat to the slow cooker with the remaining ingredients. Simmer on low for 6 to 8 hours or on high for 4 to 6 hours.

Add a couple handfuls of your favorite greens to the chili for an added veggie boost. Try chopped kale, spinach, or cabbage. Greens should be added just before serving.

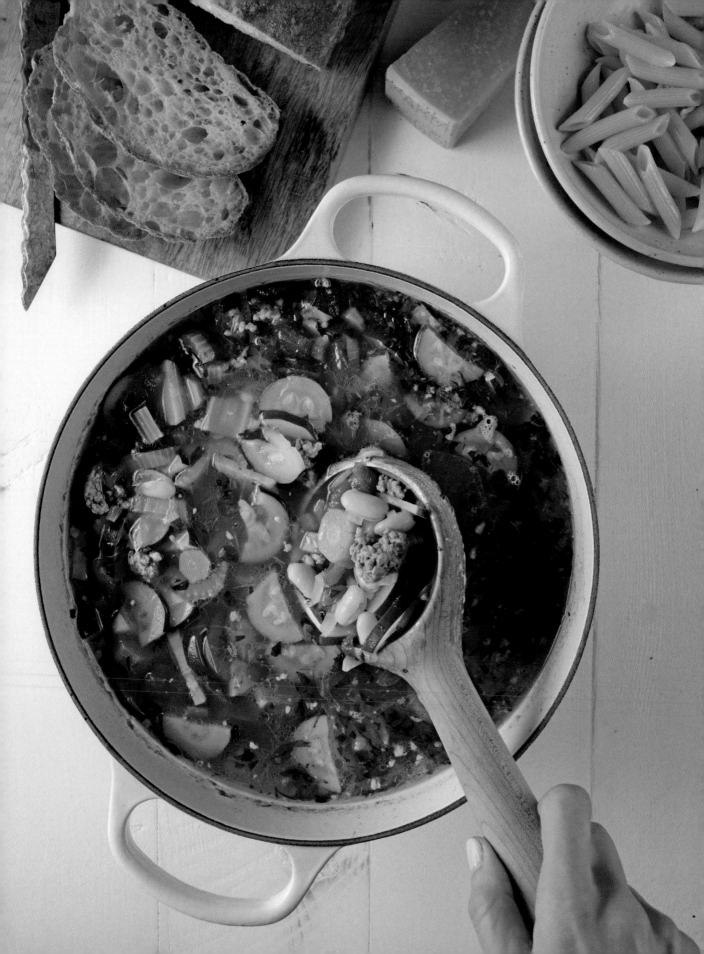

HEARTY MINESTRONE WITH SPICY SAUSAGE AND BEANS

SERVES 6

for a soup that sustains

¾ pound spicy Italian sausage meat, without casings

3 ribs celery, sliced

3 carrots, peeled and sliced

1 yellow onion, chopped

3 cloves garlic, minced

1 tablespoon minced fresh oregano or 1 teaspoon dried

1½ teaspoons fine sea salt (leave out if broth is not low-sodium)

8 cups low-sodium vegetable broth or Long Run Mineral Broth (page 111)

3 zucchinis (about 1½ pounds), halved and sliced ½ inch thick

1 can (14.5 ounces) diced tomatoes

1 can (14.5 ounces) cannellini beans, drained and rinsed, or 1½ cups cooked beans

3 cups dried penne

Freshly grated Parmesan cheese (if you have a leftover Parmesan rind, simmer it in the soup)

Minestrone, in all its veggie-loaded glory, is by far our favorite soup. Elyse has been making variations on this classic for as long as she can remember, and she recently got Shalane hooked on making it, too. Shalane likes to make a big pot of it on Sundays for replenishing postrun lunches all week long. To achieve lip-smacking flavor that doesn't require hours of simmering, we love adding a little sausage.

This soup can be made with whatever veggies (we sometimes add spinach, kale, or cabbage), beans, and meat you have on hand. We suggest following our recipe the first time you make it, but then experiment with creating your own variations thereafter.

To make this dish gluten-free, use rice pasta or quinoa pasta instead of regular pasta. To make it vegetarian, leave out the sausage and season with additional oregano, garlic, and crushed red pepper to taste.

1. Heat a large heavy-bottomed pot over medium-high heat. Add the sausage and cook, using a wooden spoon to break apart the sausage, until the meat is lightly browned, about 3 minutes.

2. Transfer the sausage to a small bowl and set aside. Pour off all but about a tablespoon of the rendered fat (or if your sausage was lean, add about a tablespoon of olive oil). Add the celery, carrots, onion, garlic, oregano, and ½ teaspoon of the salt and cook, stirring occasionally, until the vegetables are soft but not brown, about 5 minutes.

3. Add the broth, zucchini, tomatoes, beans, cooked sausage, and the remaining 1 teaspoon salt, and bring to a boil. Reduce the heat and simmer, covered, 25 to 30 minutes. Taste and season with additional salt, if needed.

4. Meanwhile, cook the pasta in a separate pot according to package directions. Drain and set aside.

5. Place a small serving of pasta (about ½ cup) in each soup bowl. Ladle the soup on top. Sprinkle with Parmesan and serve.

6. Store leftover pasta separately from leftover soup, to prevent the pasta from soaking up all the broth and turning soggy.

To get an even bigger veggie fix and load up on calcium and iron, add 3 cups chopped kale or spinach in the last 10 minutes of simmering.

FLU-FIGHTER CHICKEN AND RICE STEW

SERVES 5

for putting up a good fight

1 tablespoon extra-virgin olive oil

5 carrots, sliced

1 yellow onion, chopped

1 teaspoon fine sea salt (leave out if broth is not low-sodium)

8 cloves garlic, minced

2 tablespoons finely chopped fresh ginger

¼ to ½ teaspoon red pepper flakes (depending on spice preference)

6 cups low-sodium chicken broth or Classic Chicken Bone Broth (page 113)

1 pound boneless, skinless chicken breasts and thighs

1 cup short-grain brown rice

3 cups packed fresh spinach

1 cup chopped fresh parsley leaves

1 tablespoon fresh lemon juice

Parmesan cheese (optional)

Whether you're coming down with something, can't seem to shake a nasty cold, are suffering from digestive distress, or just want to give your immune system a boost, our stew has got your back. This soul-restoring dish is loaded with immune-boosting and anti-inflammatory ingredients including garlic, ginger, and parsley.

Our grandparents were on to something when they discovered the healing powers of chicken soup. We've taken things a step further by creating a comforting stew version of grandma's soup loaded with chicken, vegetables, and rice. A bowlful of these highly digestible ingredients will ensure your body doesn't have to work as hard to get what it needs.

For best results, use a mix of white and dark meat chicken. Not only is dark meat richer in flavor, it's also richer in muscle-building nutrients and will leave you feeling satisfied longer.

Make this dish in a slow cooker if you prefer to prep dinner in the morning and have it ready pronto after a long day of work.

1. Heat the oil in a large heavy-bottomed pot over medium-high heat. Add the carrots, onion, and salt and cook, stirring occasionally, until soft but not brown, about 5 minutes. Add the garlic, ginger, and pepper flakes and cook, stirring continuously, for 1 minute.

2. Add the broth, chicken, and rice and bring to a boil. Reduce the heat to low and simmer, covered, until the chicken is cooked through and the rice is tender, 30 minutes. Remove the chicken from the pot, place on a cutting board, and use two forks to shred it.

3. Return the chicken to the pot and stir in the spinach, parsley, and lemon juice. If too thick, thin with a little additional broth or water. Taste and season with additional salt and pepper flakes, if needed. Ladle into soup bowls and top with freshly grated Parmesan (if desired).

4. To make this dish in a slow cooker, simply combine the oil, carrots, onion, salt, garlic, ginger, pepper flakes, broth, chicken, and rice. Cook on high for 4 hours or low for 6 to 8 hours. Just before serving, add the spinach, parsley, and lemon juice and more broth if too thick.

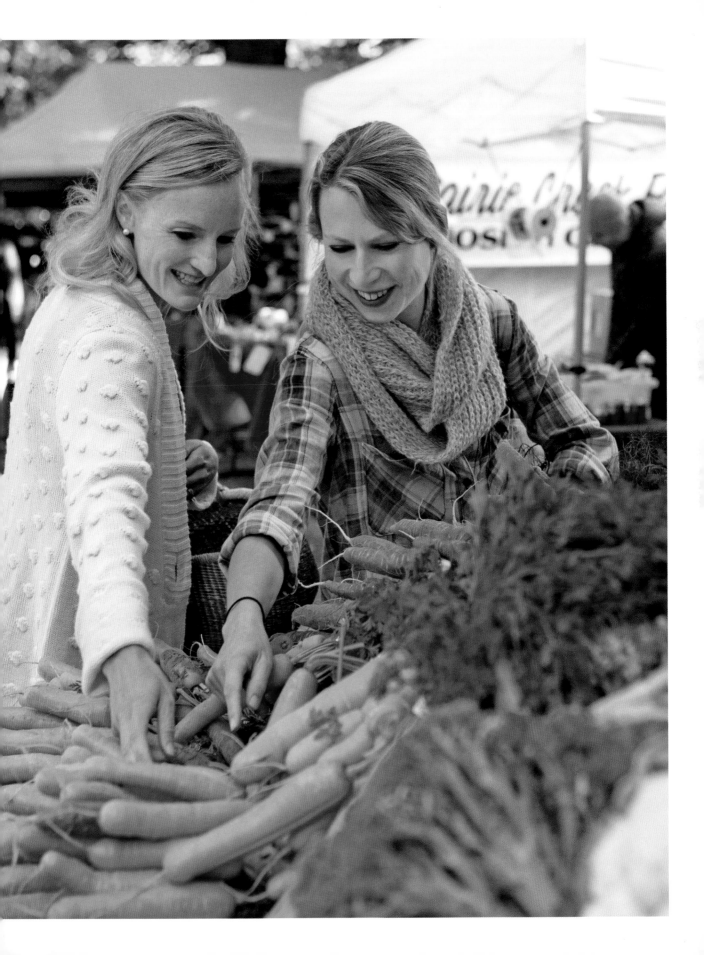

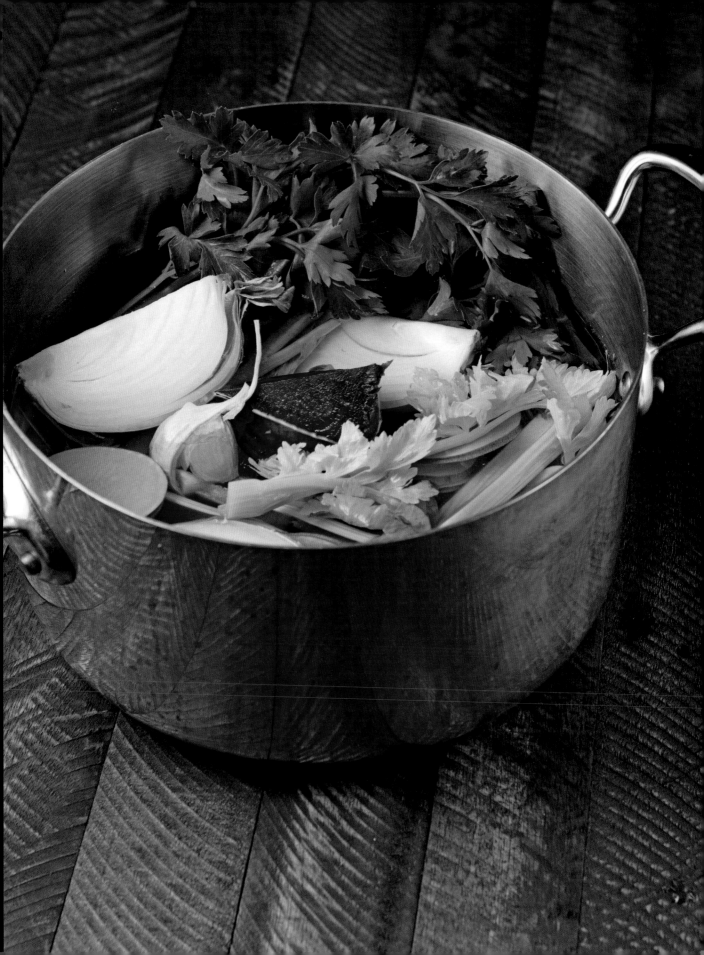

LONG RUN MINERAL BROTH

MAKES 3 QUARTS

for every ailment under the sun

If you make just one recipe in this book, let it be this one. (You'd be missing out on many memorable dishes, but at least we could sleep at night knowing you were sipping on incredibly healing nourishment!) For this recipe, we consulted with mineral-broth connoisseur and five-time cookbook author Rebecca Katz. Rebecca is a fellow graduate of the Natural Gourmet Institute and has been an influential mentor of Elyse's since Elyse's graduation from the same program. Rebecca's inspiring books include *The Cancer-Fighting Kitchen*, *The Longevity Kitchen*, and *The Healthy Mind Cookbook*.

Bone broth and vegetable broth are made by slowly simmering bones and vegetables in a large pot of water for hours until all the nutrients are extracted. Our great-grandparents used to make broths this way, but unfortunately, as our lives have sped up, this traditional food has been forgotten. Thankfully, there has been a recent revival in the art and science behind making these exceptionally nourishing tonics.

At our request, Rebecca specially crafted this recipe with a runner's needs in mind. The broth is rich in magnesium, potassium, calcium, and manganese—all essential for speeding up recovery time after a long run. A small mugful is also rich in antioxidants including vitamins A, C, E, and K. The vegetables are left unpeeled since there's a lot of power in the peel. Sip this broth straight up or use instead of store-bought broth in any of our soup recipes.

---

1 medium beet, scrubbed and cut into quarters

1 yellow onion, unpeeled and cut into quarters

3 carrots, unpeeled and cut into thirds

½ bunch celery, including the heart and leaves, cut into thirds

2 sweet potatoes, unpeeled and cut into chunks

½ bunch fresh flat-leaf parsley

5 large cloves garlic, unpeeled and smashed

1-inch knob ginger, unpeeled and sliced

8-inch strip kombu (seaweed; learn more on page 16)

6 black peppercorns

1 bay leaf

4 quarts cold filtered water

2 teaspoons fine sea salt

(continued)

1. Rinse all the vegetables well, including the kombu. Put the beet, onion, carrots, celery, sweet potatoes, parsley, garlic, ginger, kombu, peppercorns, and bay leaf in a 6-quart or larger stockpot. Add the water, cover, and bring to a boil over high heat. Reduce the heat to low and simmer, partially covered, for 1½ hours. As the broth simmers, some of the water will evaporate. Add more water if the vegetables begin to peek out. Simmer until the full richness of the vegetables can be tasted.

2. Strain the broth through a mesh sieve placed over a large heatproof container (toss or compost the veggie remains). Stir in the salt, adding more to taste if needed. Let cool to room temperature before refrigerating or freezing.

3. Store in an airtight container in the refrigerator for up to 6 days or in the freezer for up to 4 months. For individual servings, pour the broth (after cooling) into silicone muffin or ice cube trays, freeze, and transfer to gallon-size freezer bags.

 Add 1 tablespoon pasture-raised beef gelatin (we like Great Lakes Gelatin) per 8 ounces liquid to create a quick, nutrient-rich bone broth loaded with collagen. Collagen is an easy-to-digest protein that promotes joint health, maintains healthy bones, and can help reduce recovery time after a long run.

Or you can add 1½ pounds marrow bones from grass-fed organic beef (first roast the bones at 350°F for 30 minutes), or add 1 pound chicken bones (no need to roast) and 3 teaspoons apple cider vinegar or freshly squeezed lemon juice (both of which will pull the collagen out of the bones). Then increase the simmering time to 4 hours or longer.

 If you don't want to tend to the broth on the stove, you can make this recipe in a slow cooker or an Instant Pot (electric pressure cooker). In a slow cooker, simmer on high for 4 to 6 hours or low for 8 or more hours.

CLASSIC CHICKEN BONE BROTH

MAKES 4 QUARTS

for bone-building nourishment

After convincing Shalane that bone broth just might be a perfect recovery food for runners, Elyse invited Shalane over to learn how to make it. When Shalane showed up, Elyse had a pot ready for straining that had been simmering overnight. As we began pouring the broth through the strainer, Shalane shrieked and exclaimed, "Is this a witch's brew?!" For a good laugh, Elyse had tossed a couple of chicken feet into the pot. In our recipe below, the chicken feet are definitely optional.

We believe in the nourishing powers (and incredible flavor) of traditionally made bone broths. There's a reason why recipes like this one have been handed down for generations. Bone broth is a rich source of collagen, glucosamine, and minerals including calcium and magnesium, making it the perfect healing food for common running injuries like stress fractures or knee problems. It's also rich in gelatin, which can help heal the gut, boost the immune system, and fight inflammation.

The next time you roast a whole chicken (page 130), store the leftover bones in your freezer until you're ready to make broth. Or ask your butcher if he sells leftover bones or chicken backs.

Adapted from Nourishing Traditions *by Sally Fallon*

---

2 to 3 pounds chicken bones (preferably free-range)

2 chicken feet (optional . . . if you're brave)

4 quarts cold filtered water

2 tablespoons apple cider vinegar

2 yellow onions, unpeeled and cut into quarters

3 carrots, unpeeled and cut into thirds

½ bunch celery, including the heart and leaves, cut into thirds

6 black peppercorns

1 bay leaf

1 bunch fresh parsley

1. Place the chicken bones and chicken feet (if using) in a 6-quart or larger stockpot or slow cooker. Add the water and vinegar and let stand for 30 minutes.

2. Rinse all the vegetables well and add the onions, carrots, celery, peppercorns, and bay leaf to the pot or slow cooker. Bring to a boil over high heat. Reduce the heat to low and simmer, covered, for at least 8 hours and up to 24 hours (for maximum nutrient extraction). If using a slow cooker, cook on low for 24 hours. Keep an eye on the broth to ensure the bones stay fully submerged in water. Add more water if needed.

3. In the last 10 minutes of simmering, add the parsley (for an extra mineral boost!).

4. Strain the broth through a large mesh sieve placed over a large heatproof container. Discard the vegetables and bones. Transfer the broth to the fridge to cool, then skim off any fat that rises to the top.

5. If drinking the broth as a healing remedy, add sea salt or miso to taste prior to sipping. Or use as the base in our Flu-Fighter Chicken and Rice Stew (page 108) or any of our soup recipes.

6. Store in an airtight container in the refrigerator for up to 5 days or in the freezer for up to 3 months. For individual servings, pour the broth (after cooling) into silicone muffin or ice cube trays, freeze, and transfer to gallon-size freezer bags.

GARDEN GAZPACHO

SERVES 5

2 pounds tomatoes, quartered

1 cucumber, peeled and quartered

1 jalapeño chile pepper, stem removed (for a milder gazpacho, discard the seeds), wear plastic gloves when handling

4 cloves garlic

1 tablespoon soy sauce (preferably shoyu or tamari)

2 teaspoons balsamic vinegar

1 teaspoon fine sea salt

¼ teaspoon freshly ground black pepper

1 yellow bell pepper, seeded and finely chopped

1 Granny Smith apple, finely chopped

¼ red onion, finely chopped

2 tablespoons extra-virgin olive oil (optional)

¼ cup minced fresh cilantro, basil, parsley, or mint (optional)

for a mood-lifting summer soup

A chilled gazpacho soup is one of those dishes that brightens your mood as you're eating it—especially if you're slurping it on a hot summer day when your body is craving nourishing hydration. The key to an impressive gazpacho is to patiently wait until tomatoes are truly in season (better yet, grow the tomatoes in your own backyard!).

This recipe comes to us from our cookbook assistant, Natalie Bickford, who finally got her grandma to write down the family recipe for her favorite summer soup. Natalie spent her summers on her grandma's farm in Canada and has lasting memories of devouring this soup on hot days.

Bonus: Tomatoes are an excellent source of the antioxidant lycopene, which supports bone health and decreases inflammation.

1. In a high-speed blender or food processor, place the tomatoes, cucumber, chile pepper, garlic, soy sauce, balsamic vinegar, salt, and black pepper. Process on high speed until smooth.

2. Pour the soup into a large bowl with a lid. Add in the bell pepper, apple, and onion and stir to combine.

3. Place in the fridge to chill for at least 2 hours or overnight to allow the flavors to meld.

4. Stir before serving. Ladle into bowls and top each with a drizzle of oil and a sprinkle of herbs (if desired).

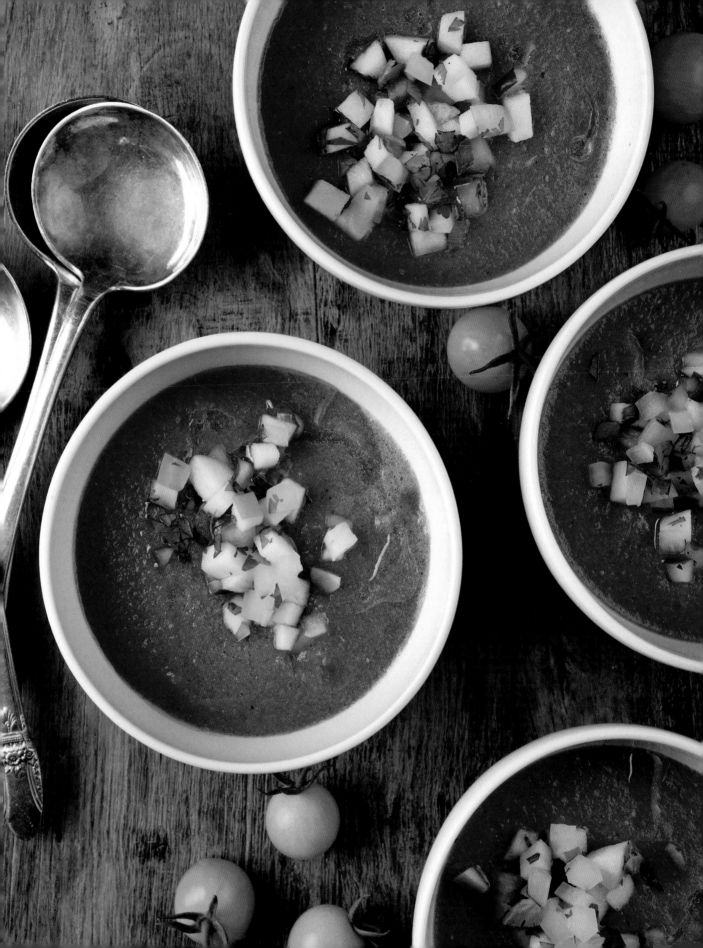

CARROT-GINGER SOUP

SERVES 4

for healing nourishment

Who knew that humble carrot soup could be so incredibly silky and rich-tasting? Since our friend Tressa Yellig, owner of the heartwarming Broth Bar in Portland, shared this recipe with us, we've been whipping up double batches. The secret to creamy bliss without the addition of heavy cream is simmering the carrots with a small amount of rice.

For the ultimate in healing nourishment, we recommend making this recipe with homemade bone broth. Learn more about our favorite mineral-rich healing tonic on page 113. To make this recipe vegan-friendly, swap the chicken broth for our Long Run Mineral Broth (page 111) and use olive oil instead of butter.

2 tablespoons unsalted butter

2 yellow onions, sliced

1½ pounds carrots, peeled and roughly chopped

1 teaspoon fine sea salt (leave out if broth is not low-sodium)

4 cups Classic Chicken Bone Broth (page 113) or store-bought low-sodium chicken broth

2 tablespoons uncooked rice (white or brown)

2 tablespoons lemon juice (1 to 2 lemons)

1 tablespoon grated fresh ginger

½ teaspoon freshly ground black pepper (optional)

1. In a large pot over medium-high heat, melt the butter. Add the onions, carrots, and salt and cook, stirring occasionally, until the vegetables soften, about 8 minutes.

2. Add the broth and rice to the pot. Bring to a boil, then reduce the heat to low. Simmer, covered, until the carrots are very tender and the rice has cooked through, 35 to 40 minutes.

3. Turn off the heat and allow the soup to cool for 10 to 15 minutes. Use a ladle to transfer the soup to a blender and process until smooth, starting on low speed and increasing slowly. Please note: Adding hot items to a blender causes the pressure to expand and can blow off the lid, so hold it firmly in place and blend on low. Alternatively, use an immersion (stick) blender.

4. Once the mixture is blended, return it to the pot and stir in the lemon juice, ginger, and pepper (if using). Taste the soup and add additional salt, if needed.

5. Warm the soup over low heat just before serving. If the soup thickens, thin with a little water until the desired consistency is reached.

MISO SOUP WITH WAKAME

SERVES 6

for pure nourishment

For a richer soup, add cooked buckwheat or soba noodles to individual bowls and top with a soft-boiled egg. Don't cook the noodles in the soup broth unless you're serving the whole pot right away, or they'll turn to mush.

We're willing to bet you always order miso soup when you go out for sushi but have never made it at home. Well, we're about to show you just how easy it is to make this nutrient-powerhouse.

Did you know? Studies show seaweed is the most nutrient-dense food on the planet. In this recipe, we use iron-rich dried wakame, which comes to life after a short simmer. And miso paste is a top-notch food for runners since it's rich in probiotics. We love food-based probiotics because they keep your gut healthy with digestion-enhancing bacteria. This ensures your body is able to extract the maximum amount of nutrients from all the amazing food you've been eating while cooking the recipes in this book!

1 tablespoon toasted sesame oil or extra-virgin olive oil

3 cloves garlic, minced

2 quarts water

2 cups thinly sliced cremini mushrooms

1 block (14 ounces) extra-firm tofu, cubed

¼ cup dried wakame flakes (seaweed; learn more on page 16)

¼ cup barley or red miso paste

1 tablespoon soy sauce (preferably tamari or shoyu)

3 scallions, finely sliced (optional)

1. Heat the oil in a large pot over medium heat. Cook the garlic, stirring frequently, until fragrant but not browning, 3 to 5 minutes.

2. Add the water, mushrooms, tofu, and wakame to the pot. Bring to a boil, then reduce the heat and simmer, covered, for 10 to 15 minutes.

3. Turn off the heat. Ladle a spoonful of broth into a small bowl. Add the miso paste and stir until fully dissolved, then pour back into the pot. Add the soy sauce. Taste and season with additional miso or soy sauce if needed.

4. Ladle into small bowls, top with scallions (if using), and serve.

TIP

It's important to remove the soup from the heat before stirring in the miso paste. High heat can kill the good bacteria in the miso.

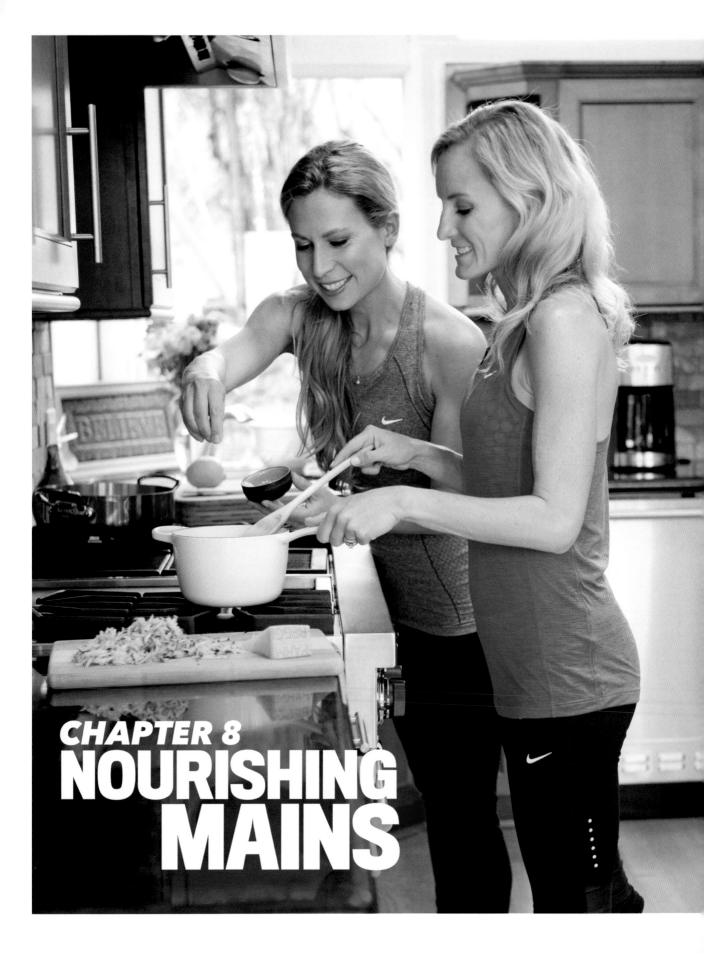

CHAPTER 8
NOURISHING MAINS

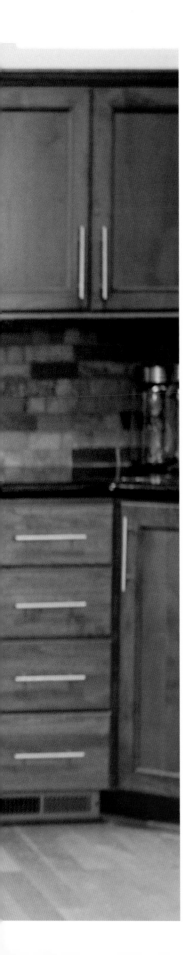

HIGH-ALTITUDE BISON MEATBALLS WITH SIMPLE MARINARA

SERVES 4

for recovery and preventing iron-deficiency

1 egg, beaten

½ cup finely grated Parmesan cheese, plus more for garnish

1 cup finely minced kale (about 4 leaves), stems discarded (a food processor works great for mincing)

¼ cup almond meal or almond flour or fine bread crumbs

3 cloves garlic, minced

1 teaspoon dried oregano

½ teaspoon fennel seeds

¾ teaspoon fine sea salt

½ teaspoon red pepper flakes

1 pound ground bison or ground beef (preferably not lean)

2 tablespoons extra-virgin olive oil

1 recipe Simple Marinara Sauce (page 171)

12 ounces dried spaghetti (gluten-free if sensitive)

8 fresh basil leaves, torn (optional)

Bison's bright red hue comes from iron, and for a runner, iron is key to keeping your red blood cells efficiently transporting oxygen to your hardworking muscles. Even a slight iron deficiency can seriously impact your energy level. Not good when you're training to break records!

These rock-star meatballs are Shalane's saving grace when training at high altitude in Flagstaff, Arizona. Bison, aka buffalo, is also high in protein and essential fatty acids, making this dish a perfect recovery meal after a 24-mile training run at 6,910 feet (or, for the sane, a 6-mile trail run!).

1. In a large bowl, stir together the egg, Parmesan, kale, almond meal, garlic, oregano, fennel seeds, salt, and pepper flakes. Add the bison (or beef) and use your hands to thoroughly combine the meat. Form the mixture into 12 meatballs, about 2 inches in diameter. Roll each meatball firmly in your hands to ensure they hold together.

2. In a large Dutch oven or wide heavy-bottomed pot with a lid, warm the oil over medium-high heat. Place the meatballs in the pot in a single layer without crowding them, and cook, turning the meatballs so they brown on all sides, about 5 minutes. Scrape the brown bits off the bottom of the pot as you go. Set the meatballs aside on a plate. (If using ground beef, pour out all but 1 to 2 tablespoons of the fat prior to making the sauce.)

3. In the same pot, make the Simple Marinara Sauce. Add the meatballs. Reduce the heat to low and simmer, uncovered, stirring occasionally, until the sauce thickens, 30 to 45 minutes. Cover and keep warm over low heat until ready to serve.

4. While the sauce is simmering, cook the pasta according to the package directions.

5. To serve, divide the pasta among 4 warmed pasta bowls and arrange the meatballs on top along with a generous ladle of sauce. Garnish with Parmesan and fresh basil, if using.

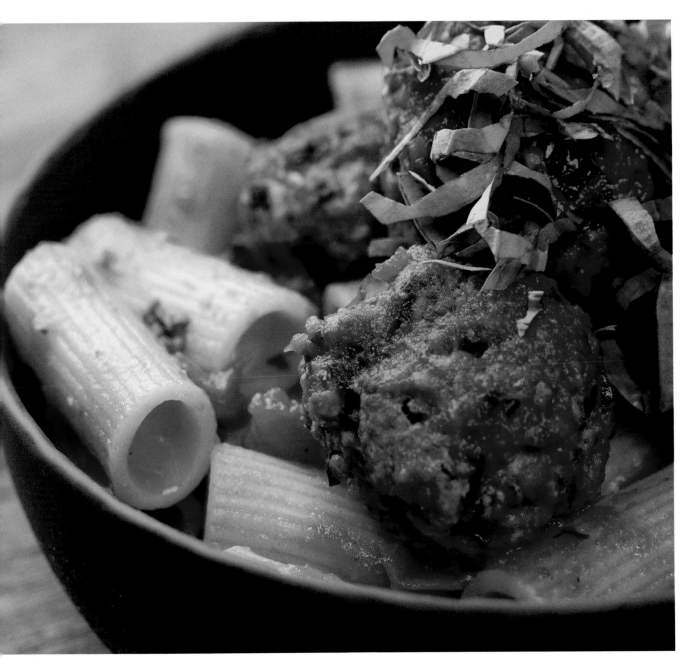

TIP

The Italians were on to something when they started
putting fennel in meat sauces. Fennel not only adds incredible
depth, but also helps us digest the fat in meat.

 Serve the meatballs and sauce on top of zucchini
noodles (see page 122) for an added veggie
boost—great for the gluten-intolerant.

In a time crunch? Skip forming the meatballs. Simply
sauté all the meatball ingredients minus the almond
meal and egg, simmer in the sauce, and serve as a
Bolognese-style sauce over pasta.

ZUCCHINI PESTO "PASTA"

SERVES 2

for a satisfying alternative to pasta

Experiment with different types of pestos made with turnip greens, beet greens, arugula, basil, or any combination and walnuts or cashews. Use the recipe on page 67 as your starting point.

Come springtime there's no better alternative to pasta than hand-cut "zoodles." And there's no better match for zucchini noodles than our Arugula Cashew Pesto (page 67).

You don't need fancy knife skills to transform a whole zucchini into noodles. A vegetable spiralizer, mandoline slicer, or good old-fashioned peeler works fabulously. (If you're on a quest to get your kids to eat more veggies, a vegetable spiralizer is a fun, worthwhile investment.)

This pasta is fab for the gluten-free crowd, but you don't have to be a strict Paleo-ite to enjoy this veggie-forward meal. Even Elyse's pasta-loving husband, Andy, gave this dish a rave review.

---

4 unpeeled zucchinis (about 2 pounds), ends discarded

2 tablespoons extra-virgin olive oil

¼ teaspoon fine sea salt

½ cup Arugula Cashew Pesto (page 67)

Freshly ground black pepper

1. Use a vegetable spiralizer, mandoline slicer, or peeler to thinly slice the entire zucchini into pasta ribbons.

2. Heat the oil in a large skillet over medium heat. Add the zucchini noodles and salt and use tongs to toss. Cook, stirring occasionally with tongs, until the zucchini begins to release its juices, 3 to 5 minutes.

3. Reduce the heat to low, stir in the pesto, and cook, tossing continuously, until the pesto melts into a sauce, 2 to 3 minutes. Taste and add salt and pepper, if needed.

4. Divide between 2 warmed pasta bowls and, if desired, top with grilled or broiled salmon or Fish en Papillote with Lemon and Olives (page 125).

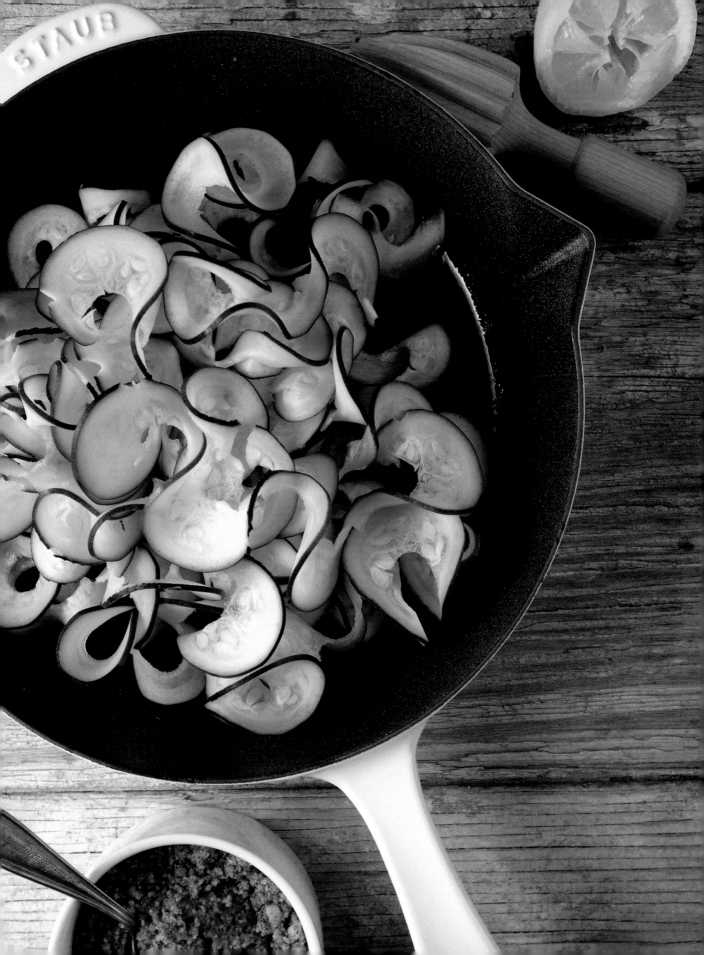

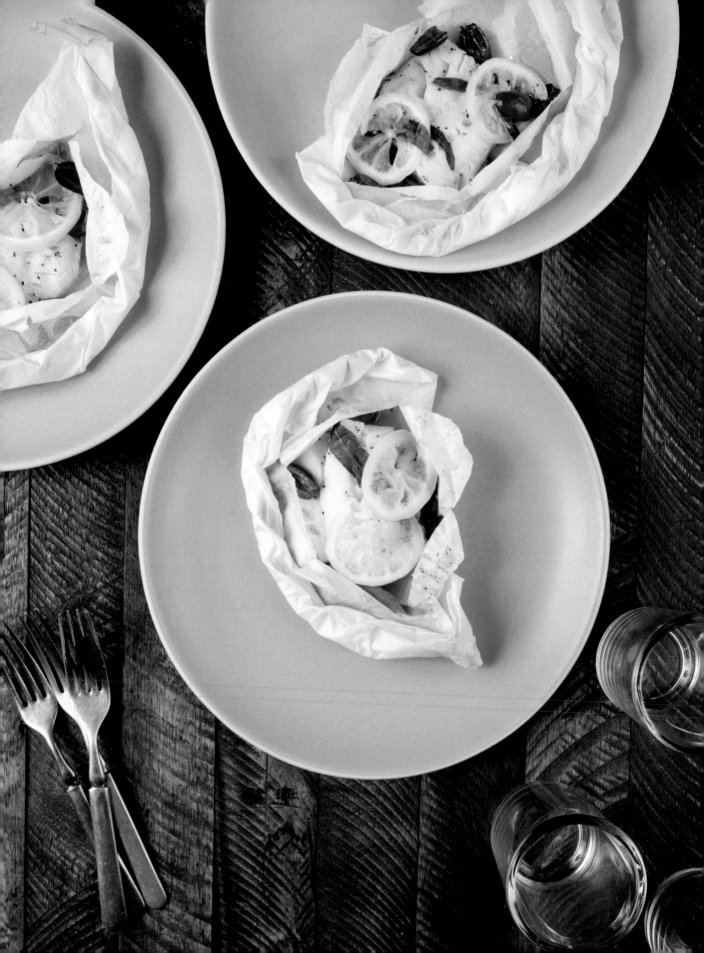

FISH EN PAPILLOTE WITH LEMON AND OLIVES

SERVES 2

for inspiring weeknight dinners

Cooking "en papillote" is a beautifully simple French technique for steam-cooking individual portions of fish in a parchment packet. By cooking the fillets in tightly sealed packets, the fish stays super moist and takes on the aroma of lemon and herbs.

We like to devour the fish right out of the packet with a hunk of crusty baguette for soaking up the flavorful juices. The best part is the aromatic burst of steam when you slit the packet open. This is fancy enough to serve to dinner guests, yet simple enough for a no-fuss weeknight dinner.

Wild local salmon is our favorite here in Oregon, but you can swap in any other healthy sustainable fillet. We highly recommend consulting SeafoodWatch.org to discover the delicious and sustainable seafood options in your area.

¾ pound favorite flaky fish, cut into 2 fillets (salmon, sole, arctic char, halibut, tilapia)

Fine sea salt

Freshly ground black pepper

1 tablespoon butter or extra-virgin olive oil

6 fresh sage leaves or 6 fresh thyme sprigs

4 thin lemon slices

¼ cup kalamata olives, pitted and sliced

1. Preheat the oven to 450°F. Tear off two 15-inch sheets of parchment paper (not waxed paper). Fold each sheet in half widthwise, then open back up, and place each fillet just in front of the crease.

2. Top each fillet with a pinch of salt and pepper. Divide the butter or oil, sage or thyme, lemon slices, and olives between the fillets.

3. Fold over the top half of the parchment paper and then tightly roll the edges from end to end to seal the fish into a packet. You don't want any steam escaping because that's what will cook the fish and keep it moist.

4. Place the packets on a rimmed baking sheet and roast in the center of the oven for 8 to 10 minutes, depending on the thickness of the fillets.

5. Transfer the packets to a plate, slit open, and eat right out of the packet with a side of roasted veggies and slices of crusty baguette (if desired). Also fantastic served alongside our Zucchini Pesto "Pasta" (page 122).

BURST CHERRY TOMATO LINGUINE WITH SHRIMP

SERVES 2

for the love of pasta

While living and working in Geneva, Switzerland, just a stone's throw away from the food mecca of Italy, Elyse was lucky enough to have the opportunity to take cooking classes in Venice, Tuscany, and Piedmont. From these classes, she gained an appreciation for seasonal simplicity. When the fruits and vegetables are picked at their peak, it takes little effort to create a swoon-worthy dish.

We make this pasta dish when the Sun Gold tomatoes in our backyard planter boxes are overtaking the rest of the garden. No sauce can beat it, and no long sweat over the stovetop is needed. The sweet little cherry tomatoes burst into a luscious sauce in 10 minutes tops.

6 ounces dried linguine or spaghetti

2 tablespoons extra-virgin olive oil, plus more for drizzling

2 pints cherry tomatoes (Sun Gold or other variety)

½ teaspoon fine sea salt

½ pound raw shrimp, peeled, deveined, and rinsed

3 cloves garlic, minced

¼ teaspoon red pepper flakes

12 fresh basil leaves, rolled and thinly sliced, plus more for garnish

½ cup grated Parmesan cheese (optional)

1. Bring a large pot of heavily salted water to a rolling boil and cook the pasta until al dente according to the package directions. Drain, set aside, and drizzle with a little olive oil to prevent clumping.

2. Heat the oil in a large skillet over medium-high heat. Add the tomatoes and salt and cook, stirring occasionally, until the tomatoes burst, 4 to 5 minutes.

3. Add the shrimp, garlic, and pepper flakes and simmer uncovered, stirring occasionally, until the sauce begins to thicken and the shrimp are opaque, about 5 minutes. Stir in the basil. Taste and add more salt and pepper flakes, if needed.

4. Divide the pasta between 2 warmed bowls and top with the sauce. Sprinkle with Parmesan and more fresh basil (if desired).

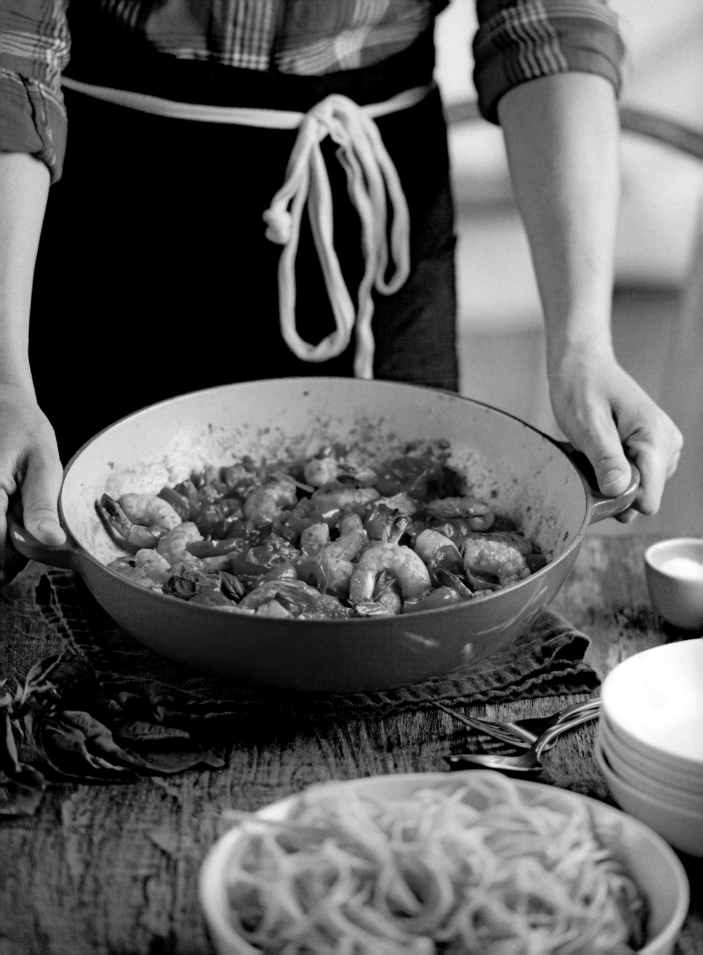

SHALANE'S BREAKFAST-MEETS-DINNER BOWL

SERVES 2

For more digestible (and flavorful) beans, make the beans from scratch. It's well worth the effort since our Spicy Black Bean recipe (page 162) makes enough for multiple dinners.

for energizing nourishment

In college, Shalane got our household hooked on topping bowls of rice with cheese-loaded scrambled eggs and any assortment of accompaniments we could dig up—the perfect solution for hungry runners on a budget. We knew we were on to something, but we never thought Shalane's Breakfast-Meets-Dinner Bowl would make it into a book someday.

Now, like us, her recipe is all grown up. We've swapped the scrambled eggs for a fried egg and Avocado Cream (page 178)—like sour cream, only better and dairy-free!—and we now prefer to make our beans from scratch (but canned beans can be used in a pinch).

This revitalizing, high-protein meal is terrific for breakfast, lunch, or dinner.

---

1 cup short-grain brown rice, rinsed

2 cups water

1 cup Spicy Black Beans (page 162) or 1 can (15 ounces) seasoned black beans

1 tablespoon olive oil

3 packed cups baby spinach or chopped kale, stems removed

¼ teaspoon fine sea salt

2 eggs

Freshly ground black pepper

Optional toppings: grated cheese, salsa, chopped tomato, chopped avocado, Avocado Cream (page 178)

1. Place the rice and water in a rice cooker or medium saucepan. Cook according to package directions or until all the water is absorbed and the rice is tender, about 20 minutes.

2. In a small saucepan with a lid, warm the beans over low heat.

3. In a nonstick pan set over medium heat, warm the oil. Add the spinach or kale and salt and cook until wilted. Set aside in a small bowl.

4. In the same pan, crack the eggs on opposite sides and season with salt and pepper. Cook the eggs "over easy" by cooking on one side until the whites set, about 2 minutes, and then flip and cook 1 minute longer (the yolk should be runny).

5. Place a serving of rice in 2 warmed bowls. Top each bowl with the beans, spinach or kale, and fried egg. Serve immediately with an assortment of your favorite toppings (if desired)—we highly recommend our Avocado Cream.

BACON-WRAPPED STUFFED CHICKEN

SERVES 4

for a hearty crowd-pleaser

Lucky for us our husbands, Steve and Andy, are good pals. They seem to agree on more than just the best spots in Portland to share a local brew. Both men on separate occasions proclaimed this dish to be their favorite. But who doesn't like a big meaty piece of chicken stuffed with cheese and encased in bacon?

Serve this chicken alongside our Sweet Potato Fries (page 161) and a simple arugula salad with our Basic Balsamic Vinaigrette (page 169), and you've got a meal fit for a celebration.

4 boneless, skinless chicken breasts

½ teaspoon fine sea salt

2 tablespoons extra-virgin olive oil

1 small yellow onion, finely chopped

1 bag (6 ounces) baby spinach (4 packed cups)

2 teaspoons dried oregano

¼ teaspoon freshly ground black pepper

1 cup crumbled feta cheese

4 slices thick-cut bacon

1. Preheat the oven to 400°F.

2. Butterfly the chicken breasts by carefully slicing them down the middle to open them up without separating the two halves. Sprinkle the chicken with about ¼ teaspoon of the salt.

3. Heat 1 tablespoon of the oil in a large skillet over medium heat. Add the onion and the remaining ¼ teaspoon salt and cook until soft but not brown, about 5 minutes. Add the spinach, oregano, and pepper and cook just until wilted. Transfer the mixture to a medium bowl and allow it to cool briefly before stirring in the cheese.

4. Place one-quarter of the spinach-cheese mixture down the middle of each chicken breast and fold over to enclose the filling. Spiral wrap 1 slice of bacon around each chicken breast and use 2 toothpicks to hold it all together.

5. In the same skillet, heat the remaining 1 tablespoon oil over medium-high heat. Place the stuffed chicken in the skillet and sear it on both sides until lightly browned, about 6 minutes.

6. Place the chicken in a ceramic baking dish (or keep it in the skillet if ovenproof). Bake in the center of the oven until a thermometer inserted in the thickest portion registers 165°F and the juices run clear, 30 to 40 minutes (cook time varies based on the size).

WHOLE ROASTED CHICKEN WITH HERBS

SERVES 4

for nourished comfort

 Don't toss out those bones. Save them in the freezer until you have time to make our seriously nourishing Classic Chicken Bone Broth (page 113).

Learning to roast a whole chicken is a rewarding experience. If you're reading this right now, then you're considering it, but probably wondering why bother when you could go out and buy an already cooked rotisserie chicken at any major grocery chain for about four bucks.

Ever wonder how those chickens can rotate in a hot case for hours and still be moist? Curious about how they can be so darn cheap? Questioning how to pronounce the list of ingredients in small print?

It's time forgo store-bought rotisserie and transform your culinary skills. With our foolproof recipe, no fancy stuffing, basting, or trussing is needed. The key is all in the bird. We recommend buying a smaller organic, free-range chicken for the juiciest results.

---

1 whole chicken (4 to 5 pounds), preferably organic and free-range

4 or 5 sprigs fresh herbs (preferably a combination of thyme, oregano, and sage)

2 tablespoons extra-virgin olive oil

1 tablespoon fine sea salt

1 teaspoon freshly ground black pepper

½ small yellow onion, cut into wedges

½ lemon, cut into wedges

3 cloves garlic, smashed

Small bunch fresh parsley

1. Preheat the oven to 450°F. Remove the giblets from the cavity of the chicken (reserve for stock) and place the chicken on a roasting pan.

2. Create a rub by mincing 1 tablespoon of the fresh herbs (thyme, oregano, sage) and combining them in a small bowl with the oil, salt, and pepper.

3. Stuff the cavity of the chicken with the onion, lemon, garlic, parsley, and any remaining sprigs of fresh herbs that will fit. Pull the skin to cover the opening.

4. Cover the chicken on all sides and crevices with the herb rub and place breast side up in the roasting pan. Fold the wing tips underneath the chicken.

5. Cook until a thermometer inserted in the inner thigh registers 165°F and the juices run clear, 1 hour. For best results, do not open the oven to check on the chicken until the hour mark. A 6- to 8-pound chicken will take longer, about 1 hour 30 minutes. Let rest for 15 minutes before carving.

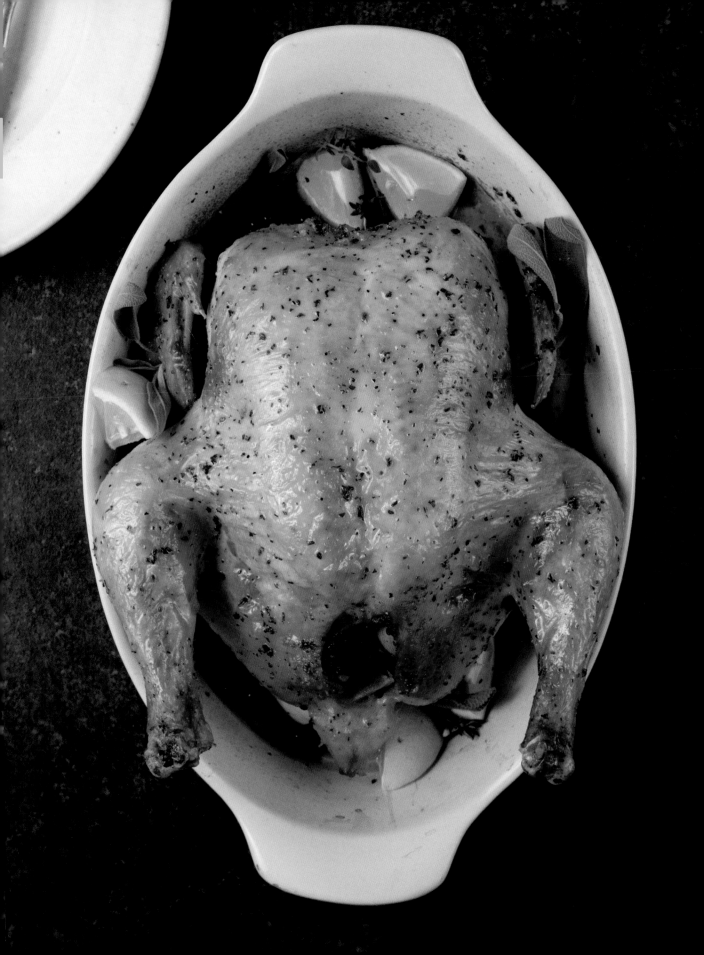

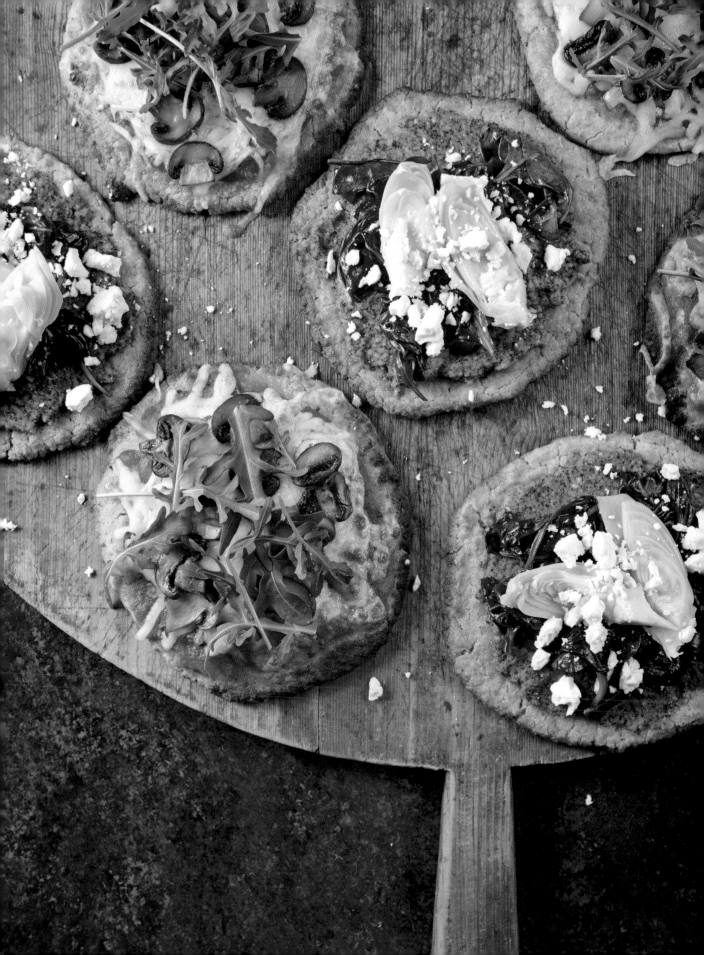

MILLET PIZZA PIES

MAKES SIX 6-INCH PIES

for gluten-free pizza bliss

Call us crazy but we like our gluten-free millet pizza crust better than regular pizza crust. It's flavorful, thin, and crispy and has serious staying power thanks to the protein-loaded combo of whole grains and beans. Also this knead-free, flour-free dough is less fussy than regular pizza dough—no dough-slinging skills needed.

On pizza night, we like to roll out a topping bar and let everyone build their own mini pies. For inspiration, see our two favorite vegetarian combos on page 134.

The crust crumbles easily, so it's best for making individual-size pizza pies and should be eaten hot right out of the oven. If you're cooking for one, don't cook all the dough at once. The uncooked batter can be stored covered in the fridge for up to 3 days or frozen for up to 3 months and thawed prior to baking.

---

1 cup millet (whole, not flour)

2 tablespoons olive oil, plus more for brushing and drizzling

1 can (15 ounces) cannellini beans, rinsed and drained, or 1½ cups cooked beans

2 eggs

1½ tablespoons white miso (learn more on page 117)

1 teaspoon dried oregano

1 teaspoon fennel seeds

1. Rinse the millet in a fine mesh sieve and drain thoroughly. In a medium saucepan over medium heat, dry-toast the millet, stirring constantly, until fragrant, about 5 minutes. Slowly add 2 cups water and bring to a boil. Reduce the heat to low, cover, and simmer until all the water is absorbed and you no longer see individual grains, 20 minutes. (You want the millet to be slightly overcooked so that it has a thick, doughy consistency. If it's still moist, simmer uncovered for a couple of minutes.) Transfer to a large bowl to cool.

2. Preheat the oven to 450°F. Line 2 baking sheets with parchment paper. Brush the parchment paper with olive oil.

3. Use a paper towel to dry the beans. In a food processor or high-speed blender, place the millet, beans, eggs, miso, oil, oregano, and fennel. Process on high until smooth and well-combined, stopping as needed to scrape down the sides and underneath the blade with a rubber spatula.

4. Use a ½-cup measuring cup to scoop an individual-size serving of dough onto a baking sheet. Use the back of a spoon to spread out and shape the dough into a thin 6-inch crust. Repeat with the remaining dough until you have 6 pies spaced out on the baking sheets. Drizzle the tops with oil.

(continued)

5. Bake in the center and lower racks of the oven for 15 minutes. Remove from the oven and use a metal spatula to carefully flip each crust. Return to the oven until the tops begin to brown, 8 minutes.

6. Top each crust with your favorite pizza toppings and return to the oven until the cheese melts, 5 minutes.

Pesto Pizza with Spinach and Artichokes

1 tablespoon extra-virgin olive oil

1 bag (6 ounces) baby spinach (4 packed cups)

¼ teaspoon fine sea salt

½ cup pesto or Arugula Cashew Pesto (page 67)

1 recipe Millet Pizza Pies (page 133)

½ cup quartered artichoke hearts

1 cup crumbled feta cheese

1. Preheat the broiler.

2. In a large skillet, heat the oil and add the spinach and salt. Cook, stirring frequently, until wilted, about 1 minute.

3. Spread the pesto in a thin layer on top of each baked pizza pie. Top each with the spinach and artichokes and sprinkle the cheese over top.

4. Place on the top rack of the oven and broil until the cheese melts, 1 to 2 minutes (keep a close eye on it to prevent burning).

Marinara Pizza with Mushrooms and Arugula

1 tablespoon olive oil

2½ cups sliced cremini or white button mushrooms

¼ teaspoon fine sea salt

1 cup marinara sauce or Simple Marinara Sauce (page 171)

1 recipe Millet Pizza Pies (page 133)

1 cup grated mozzarella or other favorite cheese

2 cups loosely packed arugula

1. Preheat the broiler.

2. In a large skillet, heat the oil and add the mushrooms and salt. Cook, stirring frequently, until soft, about 5 minutes.

3. Spread the marinara sauce in a thin layer on top of each baked pizza pie. Top each with the mushrooms and sprinkle the cheese over top.

4. Place on the top rack of the oven and broil until the cheese melts, 1 to 2 minutes (keep a close eye on the pizza to prevent burning). Top with the arugula and serve.

PENNE WITH ROASTED BUTTERNUT SQUASH AND SAGE BROWN BUTTER

SERVES 4

for devouring fall flavors

🕐 Chopping a winter squash takes serious muscle. Some grocery stores sell freshly cut butternut, which will save you time.

When the weather starts to turn cool and the days get shorter, you'll find yourself craving richer comfort foods. This pasta dish will hit the spot. For a warming, unexpected boost, we like to add a couple pinches of cinnamon to bring out the natural sweetness of the butternut.

Come summertime, swap out the butternut squash for summer squash (and leave out the cinnamon). When we grill summer favorites like zucchini, yellow squash, eggplant, and asparagus, we always grill extra to toss into simple pasta dishes like this one.

Be careful not to tell your teammates what you're making for dinner or they'll all be knocking at your door.

1 small butternut squash (about 2 pounds), peeled, halved lengthwise, seeded, and cut into ½-inch cubes

1 tablespoon extra-virgin olive oil

1 teaspoon fine sea salt

½ teaspoon freshly ground black pepper

12 ounces dried penne, ziti, or spaghetti

1 recipe Sage Brown Butter (page 172)

¼ teaspoon ground cinnamon

¼ cup grated Parmesan cheese

½ cup toasted chopped walnuts (optional)

1. Preheat the oven to 400°F.

2. Place the squash on a rimmed baking sheet and toss with the oil, ½ teaspoon of the salt, and ¼ teaspoon of the pepper. Spread out in a single layer and roast until soft and lightly browned, 30 to 40 minutes, stirring every 15 minutes.

3. When the squash is nearly done, cook the pasta according to the package directions in generously salted water. Reserve ½ cup of the pasta water, then drain and set aside.

4. Warm the butter in a large skillet over low heat. Add the squash, cinnamon, and the remaining ½ teaspoon salt and ¼ teaspoon pepper. Add the pasta water a little at a time. Add the cooked pasta and toss until the pasta is heated through and combined with the other ingredients. Taste and add additional salt and pepper, if needed.

5. Serve immediately topped with the Parmesan and walnuts (if using).

FISH TACOS WITH MANGO-AVOCADO SALSA

SERVES 4

for summer entertaining

Put on your fancy pants and serve our Garden Gazpacho (page 114) as a starter before the tacos make their grand entrance.

Being that mangos and avocados are two of Shalane's true loves, our cookbook wouldn't be complete without a mango-avocado salsa. And nothing pairs better with a sweet, creamy, and spice-kissed salsa than delectable fish tacos.

Topping each taco with a spoonful of this vibrant salsa allows you to keep the seasoning on the fish simple—just a drizzle of olive oil and a dusting of salt and pepper will do. This means you can get a refreshing summer dinner on the table in under 30 minutes.

SALSA

1 ripe mango, chopped

1 ripe avocado, chopped

1 jalapeño chile pepper, stem removed, finely chopped (include the seeds for spice), wear plastic gloves when handling

1 clove garlic, minced

¼ cup chopped cilantro

¼ teaspoon fine sea salt

¼ teaspoon freshly ground black pepper

1 to 2 tablespoons lime juice

TACOS

1 pound Pacific cod, halibut, rockfish, or wild salmon

1 tablespoon extra-virgin olive oil

1 teaspoon coarse sea salt

¼ teaspoon freshly ground black pepper

8 stone-ground corn tortillas (6-inch diameter)

1 lime, cut into wedges

8 sprigs cilantro (optional)

1. **To make the salsa:** In a medium bowl, combine the mango, avocado, chile pepper, garlic, cilantro, salt, pepper, and 1 tablespoon of the lime juice. Taste and add another tablespoon of lime juice if needed.

2. **To make the tacos:** Season the fish with the oil, salt, and pepper and allow it to come up to room temperature by leaving it out for 15 minutes. Preheat the grill to medium-high.

3. Place the fish on the grill skin side down and grill for 2 to 3 minutes, depending on the thickness of the fish. Use a metal spatula to carefully flip the fish. Grill on the second side until the fish is cooked through and no longer translucent in the middle, 2 to 3 minutes.

4. Alternatively, the fish can be cooked in the oven. Preheat the broiler. Place the fish on a foil-lined baking sheet and set it on the top rack of the oven. Broil the fish until lightly charred and no longer translucent in the middle, 3 to 5 minutes per side.

5. Transfer the fish to a clean plate, remove the skin, and use a fork to flake into bite-size pieces.

6. Fill each tortilla with the fish and a generous spoonful of the salsa. Garnish each plate with a lime wedge and the cilantro sprigs (if using).

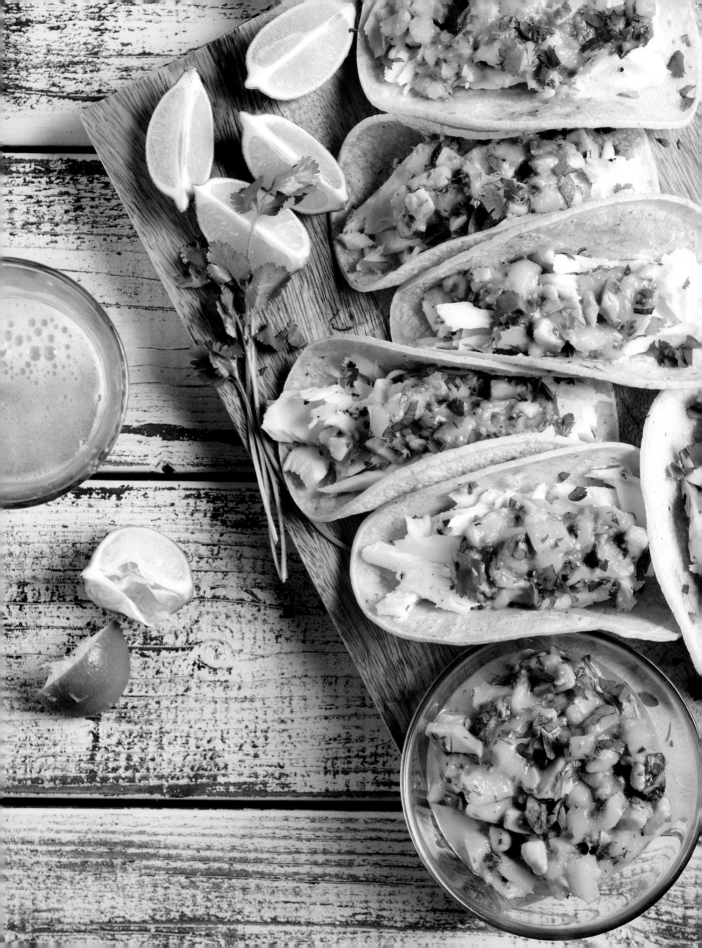

GREEK BISON BURGERS

SERVES 4

for pumping iron

For a gluten-free alternative to buns, serve the burgers between 2 slices of grilled eggplant rounds. Simply slice 1 large eggplant into 1-inch-thick slices, brush with olive oil, sprinkle with sea salt, and grill for 3 to 4 minutes per side.

These burgers are our jam. In the summer, we make them on a near weekly basis. Combining the ground meat with egg, feta, almond flour, and Greek-inspired seasonings results in the juiciest and most flavorful burgers you'll ever eat.

Shalane loves to make them with ground bison (buffalo) when training at high altitude for the iron-rich kick, but they're also foolproof made with ground beef, lamb, or turkey.

This recipe is simple enough to double or triple when feeding a crowd (Elyse multiplied the recipe by 8 for her daughter's first birthday).

---

1 egg

½ cup crumbled feta cheese

¼ cup almond flour or almond meal

1 tablespoon minced fresh oregano leaves or 1 teaspoon dried

2 cloves garlic, minced

¼ teaspoon fine sea salt

¼ teaspoon freshly ground black pepper

1 pound ground bison (buffalo) or ground beef, lamb, or turkey

4 whole wheat pitas or hamburger buns (see gluten-free substitute above), optional

Optional toppings: Avocado Cream (page 178), Chipotle Hummus (page 70), or Don't Get Beet Hummus (page 73)

1. Preheat the grill to medium-high.

2. In a large mixing bowl, combine the egg, feta, almond flour or meal, oregano, garlic, salt, and pepper. Add the meat and use your hands to combine, being careful not to overwork the meat. Form into 4 equal-size patties about 1 inch thick.

3. Grill the burgers, flipping once, until a thermometer inserted in the center registers 160°F and the meat is no longer pink, 3 or 4 minutes per side. In the last minute, warm the pitas or buns on the grill (if using).

4. Split the pitas or buns open, stuff each with a burger, and top (if desired) with a spoonful of Avocado Cream, Chipotle Hummus, or Don't Get Beet Hummus.

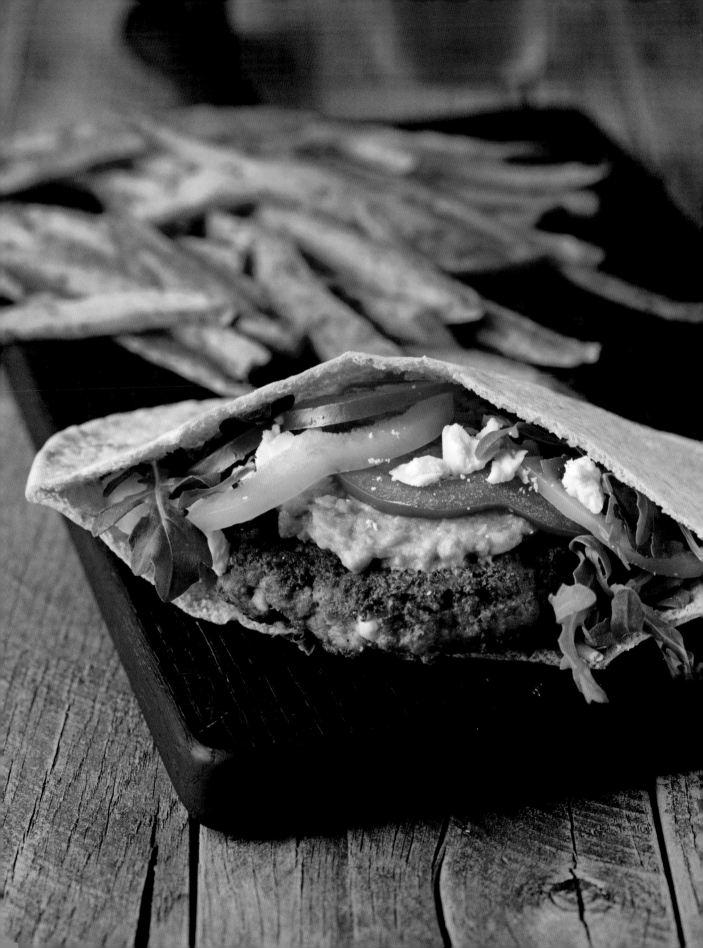

MARATHON LASAGNA

SERVES 10

for feeding a team of hungry runners

This is the dish to make when you need to feed an army of hungry runners. Hearty layers of meat, cheese, sauce, and veggies sandwiched between thick noodles—lasagna is comfort food at its best.

Our Marathon Lasagna was inspired by what Shalane eats the night before the Boston Marathon. The athlete dinner she attends every year is like Thanksgiving, complete with roasted turkey, sweet potatoes, veggies, and rolls—super nourishment to power her through 26.2 grueling miles. So we decided to create a dish that combines all this goodness and then some, and our sweet potato, spinach, and turkey lasagna was born.

The key to transforming lasagna from good to great is to season every component, so we warn you, this dish takes time. But the end result will feed a team or keep your family well fed for days (see the note below about freezing the leftovers).

We recommend making the sauce and baking the sweet potatoes the day before. And we suggest baking extra sweet potatoes so that you can whip up a batch of Sweet Potato Breakfast Cookies (page 56). Ready, set, go!

2 tablespoons olive oil

1½ pounds ground turkey

3 cloves garlic, minced

1 teaspoon dried oregano

1 teaspoon fennel seeds

¼ teaspoon red pepper flakes

1 teaspoon fine sea salt

6 cups Simple Marinara Sauce (page 171) or jarred marinara

1 pound no-boil lasagna noodles

1 bag (12 ounces) baby spinach (8 packed cups)

2 cups mashed cooked sweet potato (see note opposite)

1 container (16 ounces) whole-milk ricotta

2 eggs, beaten

¼ teaspoon freshly ground black pepper

1 pound mozzarella cheese, thinly sliced

1 cup grated Parmesan cheese

Lasagna is a genius dish to freeze for future dinners. Simply slice leftovers into individual portions, wrap tightly in foil, and freeze for up to 3 months. Place individual foil packets on a baking sheet and reheat in the oven at 350°F for 35 to 45 minutes.

1. Preheat the oven to 400°F. Place a 13 x 9 x 2-inch baking dish on top of a rimmed baking sheet.

2. Heat 1 tablespoon of the oil in a large saucepan over medium-high heat. Add the turkey, garlic, oregano, fennel, red pepper, and ½ teaspoon of the salt and cook, stirring frequently, until the turkey is lightly browned, about 5 minutes. Add the marinara sauce and simmer over low heat while preparing the remaining ingredients.

3. In a large skillet, heat the remaining 1 tablespoon oil over medium heat and cook the spinach with the remaining ½ teaspoon salt until wilted, about 3 minutes.

4. In a medium bowl, combine the sweet potato, ricotta, eggs, and black pepper.

5. In the bottom of the baking dish, spread 1½ cups of the meat sauce and top with a layer of 5 noodles. Spread half the sweet potato mixture over the noodles and top with all of the spinach. Start another layer with 1½ cups of sauce, then half the mozzarella slices, 5 noodles, and the remaining sweet potato mixture. Top with another 1½ cups of the sauce, 5 noodles, the remaining 1½ cups sauce, the remaining mozzarella slices, and finally the Parmesan.

6. Cover the dish with foil. Bake in the center of the oven on top of the baking sheet (to catch any drippings) for 25 to 30 minutes. (If you made the meat sauce and sweet potatoes in advance and they were added cold, then bake for an extra 15 minutes.) Remove the foil and bake until golden and bubbling, 10 to 15 minutes. Cool for 15 minutes prior to slicing and serving.

NOTE: To cook sweet potatoes, wrap individually in foil and bake at 400°F for 45 to 60 minutes. About 2½ pounds of uncooked sweet potatoes will make 2 cups of mashed sweet potatoes.

WILD SALMON SWEET POTATO CAKES

SERVES 4

for balanced energy

¼ cup plus 2 tablespoons virgin coconut oil

1 medium yellow onion, finely diced

¾ teaspoon fine sea salt

2 or 3 cloves garlic, minced

1 cup orange-fleshed sweet potato (yam) puree (see page 56 for instructions)

8 ounces wild salmon, skin and pin bones removed, flesh finely chopped (ask your butcher to do this)

2 eggs, beaten

½ cup almond flour

½ cup minced fresh parsley

2 tablespoons lemon juice

1 tablespoon Dijon mustard

1 teaspoon ground cumin

¼ teaspoon freshly ground black pepper

1 lemon, cut into wedges (optional)

Avocado Cream (page 178), optional

The cakes can be made ahead and arranged in an airtight container between sheets of parchment paper. Refrigerate for up to 3 days or freeze for up to 3 months. Thaw in the refrigerator before reheating at 250°F until heated through, about 20 minutes.

Instead of using worthless fillers like breadcrumbs or stale crackers, we pack our savory salmon cakes with sweet potatoes—a nutrient-dense and delicious root vegetable. These cakes are a balanced, all-in-one meal, combining a powerhouse of complete proteins, complex carbohydrates, and healthy fats.

Frying the cakes in a generous amount of coconut oil guarantees an enticing exterior and a melt-in-your-mouth center. Don't fear the fat. Coconut oil is anti-inflammatory and highly digestible—fuel that your body will use now rather than store for later.

1. In a 12-inch cast-iron skillet or heavy-bottom pan, heat 2 tablespoons of the oil over medium-high heat. Add the onion and ¼ teaspoon of the salt and cook, stirring occasionally, until the onion is soft but not brown, about 5 minutes. Add the garlic and cook, stirring constantly, for 1 minute.

2. In a bowl with the sweet potato puree, combine the onion mixture, salmon, eggs, almond flour, parsley, lemon juice, mustard, cumin, pepper, and the remaining ½ teaspoon salt.

3. Preheat the oven to 250°F. Line a baking sheet with a double layer of paper towels.

4. Wipe out the pan you cooked the onions in, then add the ¼ cup oil and warm over medium heat. When the oil begins to shimmer but is not smoking, scoop ¼ cup of the salmon batter and gently tap upside down on the side of the pan to slide the batter into the oil. Use a spatula to press down slightly so the cakes are about 1 inch thick. Cook until nicely browned on the bottom, about 3 minutes (if they're browning too quickly, turn the heat down). Carefully flip each cake over and cook until the bottoms are deeply golden and cooked through, about 2 to 3 minutes.

5. Transfer the salmon cakes to the baking sheet. Keep warm in the oven while you fry the remaining cakes. If needed, carefully wipe the skillet clean and add more oil.

6. To serve, arrange the salmon cakes on individual plates. Garnish with the lemon wedges and top with a scoop of Avocado Cream (if using).

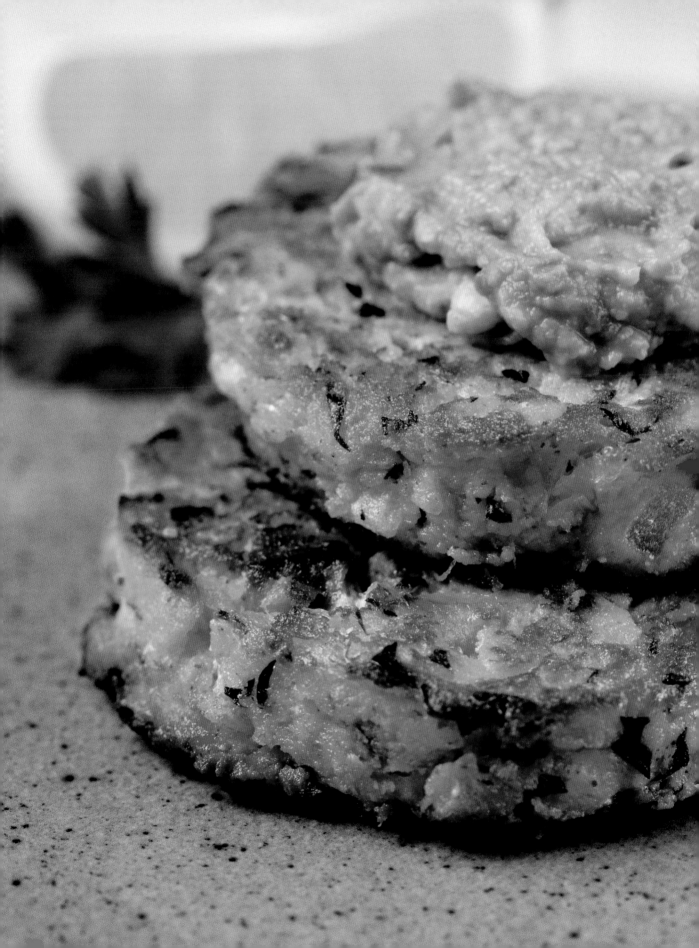

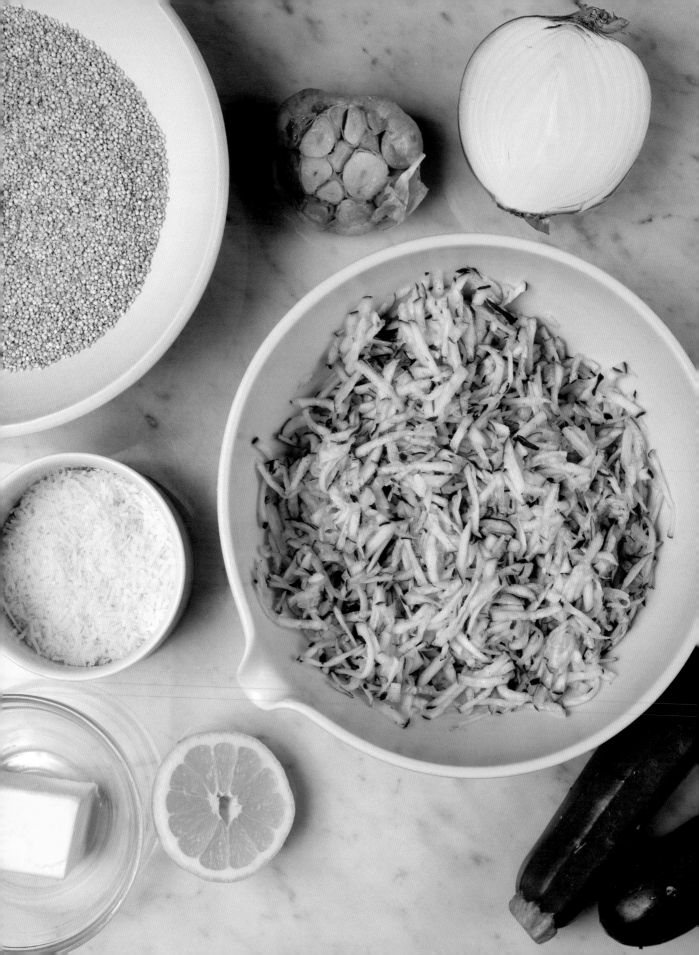

ZUCCHINI QUINOTTO WITH ROASTED GARLIC

SERVES 6

for a vegetarian feast

Forget macaroni and cheese! Risotto is the comfort food of choice in Elyse's home. After traveling to Santiago, Chile, for work, Elyse's husband, Andy, came home thrilled to report that in Chile they make risotto with quinoa and aptly call it *quinotto*.

Quinoa is a tiny protein-packed seed with global status but humble beginnings. It originates in South America, where it has been eaten for centuries in the Andes. Traditionally *quinotto* is made with heavy cream, which can be hard on a runner's digestive system. Using the magic of grated zucchini, roasted garlic, and Parmesan, Elyse was able to create a version that won't slow you down.

3 cups low-sodium vegetable or chicken broth or Classic Chicken Bone Broth (page 113)

2 tablespoons unsalted butter

1 yellow onion, diced

½ teaspoon fine sea salt

2 cups quinoa, rinsed and drained well

½ cup dry white wine

4 zucchinis (about 2 pounds), grated

1 bulb Roasted Garlic (page 75), cloves removed and mashed

1 cup grated Parmesan cheese

Grated zest of 1 lemon

2 tablespoons lemon juice

¼ teaspoon freshly ground black pepper

6 fresh basil leaves, thinly sliced (optional)

1. In a medium saucepan, bring the broth to a simmer, then turn off the heat and cover.

2. Melt the butter in a large skillet over medium heat. Add the onion and salt and cook, stirring occasionally, until soft but not brown, about 5 minutes.

3. Add the quinoa and cook, stirring continuously, until toasted (the grains will begin to crackle). Add the wine and stir until most of the moisture evaporates.

4. Ladle 1 cup of the broth over the quinoa, add the zucchini and garlic, and stir continuously until the zucchini softens, 5 to 10 minutes.

5. Reduce the heat to low. Once the moisture from the zucchini evaporates, continue adding ½ cup of the broth at a time, if needed, stirring continuously, until the quinoa is cooked through, about 10 minutes. You'll know it's ready when the individual grains open, exposing a tiny tail. Depending on how much moisture your zucchini releases, you may not need all the broth.

6. Add the Parmesan, lemon zest and juice, and pepper and stir to combine. Once the Parmesan melts, taste and add more salt and pepper, if needed.

7. Serve immediately topped with fresh basil (if using).

FIG AND PIG QUICHE

SERVES 6

for love at first bite

CRUST

1½ cups whole wheat pastry flour or all-purpose flour

½ teaspoon fine sea salt

8 tablespoons (1 stick) unsalted butter, cut into cubes and chilled in the freezer for 10 minutes

¼ to ½ cup cold water

QUICHE

8 eggs, beaten

½ cup crumbled feta cheese

¼ teaspoon fine sea salt

¼ teaspoon freshly ground black pepper

3 slices bacon, chopped

1 yellow onion, chopped

2 cups chopped kale, stems removed

4 fresh figs, stems removed, quartered, or ½ ripe pear, sliced thin

We put this recipe in the book because we want to inspire you to make your own pie crusts from scratch. Sure, store-bought refrigerated pie dough tastes half decent, but one look at the paragraph of alarming ingredients and you'll be running for the woods—partially hydrogenated lard, ferrous sulfate, potassium sorbate, and yellow 5, to name a few foes.

Meanwhile, our homemade crust contains four simple ingredients that you probably already have on hand: flour, butter, salt, and water. It's all you need to create a perfect crust for our showstopping, mile-high quiche, which combines seasonal fresh figs with smoky bacon. This is no dainty quiche. We've packed it with all our favorites, so to prevent overflow use a pie dish, which has higher sides than a traditional tart or quiche pan.

Fig season happens only twice per year, once in June and once in September, so earmark this recipe and your calendar. When figs are not available, decorate the quiche with thin slices of pear. The pie dough can be made up to 3 days in advance and kept in the fridge or frozen for up to 3 months.

1. **To make the crust:** Whisk together the flour and salt in a large mixing bowl. Use a pastry blender to cut the butter into the flour until it forms pea-size crumbles. Alternatively, a food processor can be used to combine the butter and flour into crumbles.

2. Sprinkle the water into the mixture starting with ¼ cup, then 1 tablespoon at a time while stirring, until the flour begins to come together. (If using a food processor, add the water directly and pulse briefly between additions just until the dough begins to clump.) Use your hands to shape into a ball, then flatten slightly, wrap in plastic, and chill in the fridge for at least 30 minutes.

3. Preheat the oven to 425°F with a rack set on the middle shelf.

4. On a lightly floured work surface, use a rolling pin to roll the dough into a 13-inch circle. Rotate the dough often while rolling it out to prevent it from sticking. Add more flour if needed.

(continued)

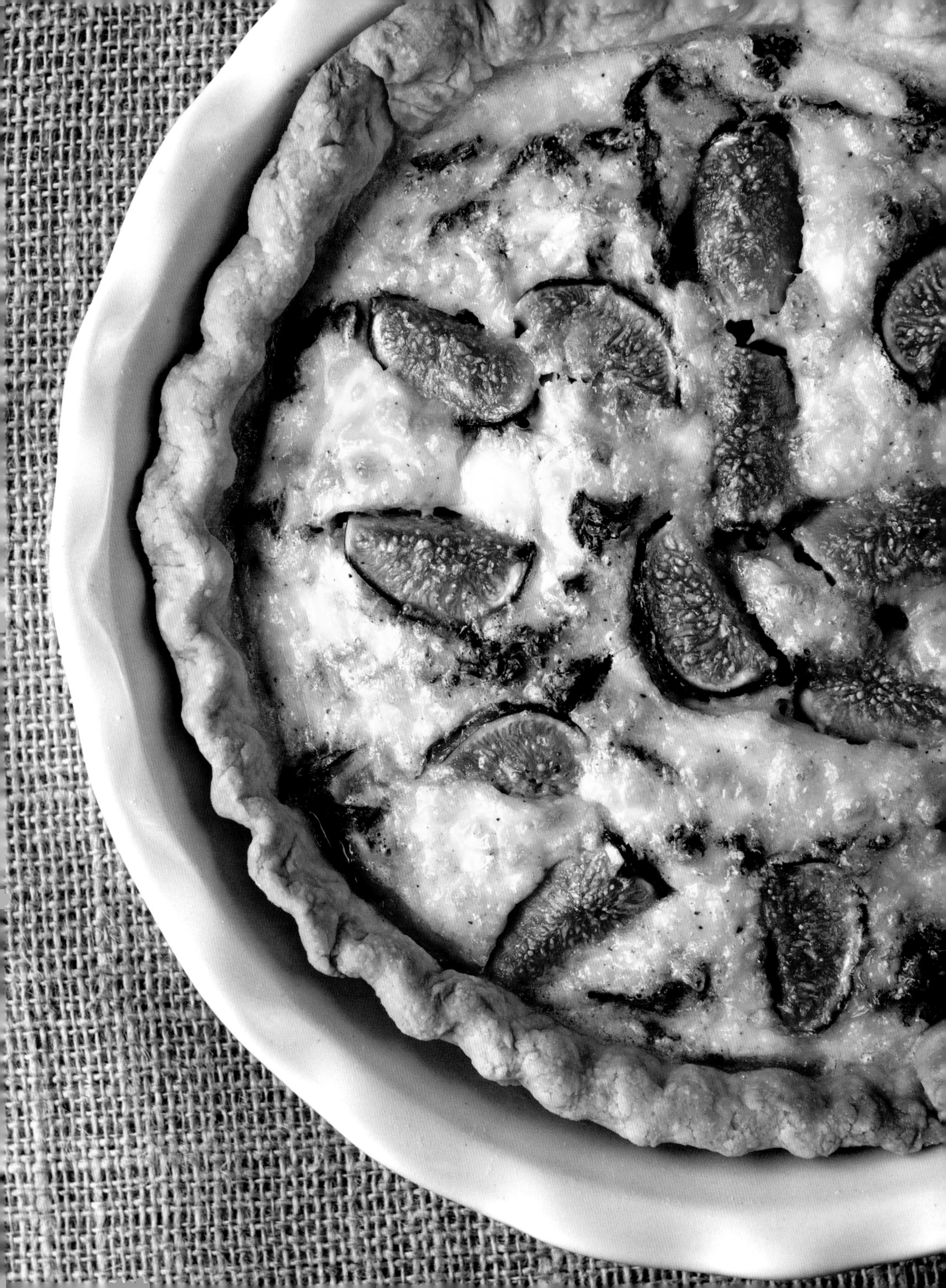

Quiche can be served any time of day. We like to serve it for dinner with a simple green salad.

To save time or to make the recipe gluten-free, this quiche can be baked without the crust, which technically means you've just created an enticing frittata.

To make this recipe vegetarian, cook the onions in 1 to 2 tablespoons olive oil instead of the bacon and add ¼ teaspoon salt.

5. Lay the crust centered in a deep 9-inch pie dish (ceramic or metal bakes better than glass). Fold any overhang under and use your fingers to crimp the edges. Prick the bottom several times with a fork. Lay a piece of parchment paper large enough to cover the entire crust over the top and weigh it down with pie weights or a cup of dry beans (this prevents the crust from collapsing).

6. Bake the crust for 20 minutes. Remove the parchment paper and pie weights or beans (discard the beans), and return the crust to the oven until lightly golden on the bottom, 8 minutes. Set the pie dish on a wire rack until ready to fill.

7. **To fill the quiche:** Reduce the oven temperature to 350°F.

8. In a medium bowl, whisk together the eggs, feta, salt, and pepper.

9. Heat a skillet over medium heat. Add the bacon and onion and cook, stirring occasionally, until lightly browned, about 5 minutes. Add the kale and cook, stirring frequently, just until wilted, about 1 minute.

10. Place the onion-kale mixture in the crust and spread it out evenly. Pour the egg mixture over top. Arrange the figs or pear on top.

11. Place the quiche in the center of the oven and bake until the eggs are set and the top is golden, 50 to 60 minutes.

12. Transfer the quiche to a wire rack and let it cool for 10 to 15 minutes. Run a knife around the edge to loosen, cut into 6 slices, and serve immediately.

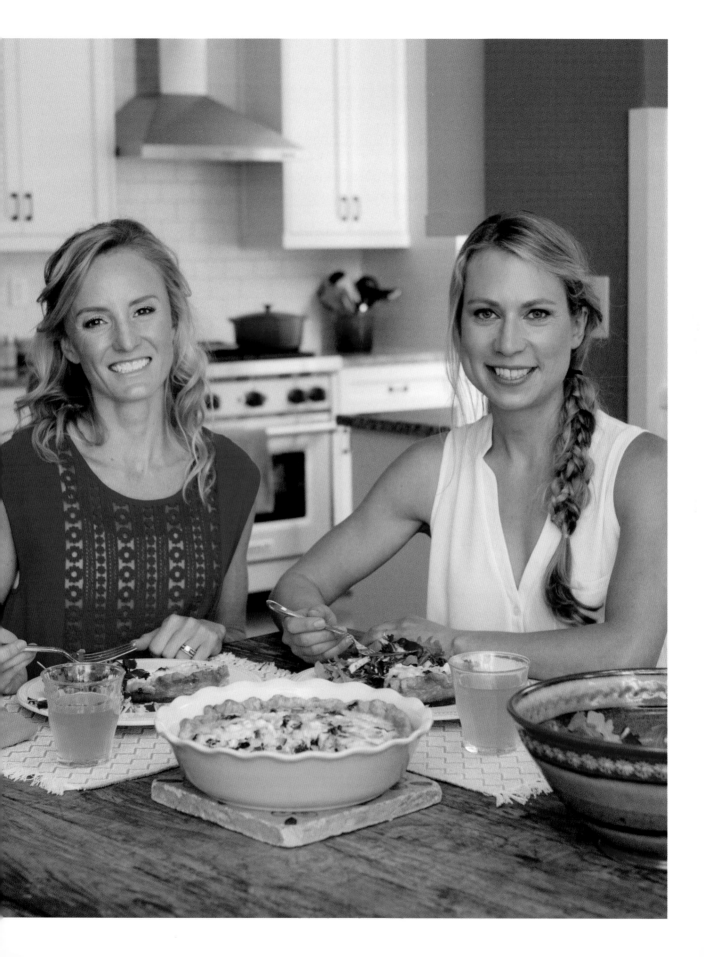

PARMESAN AND HERB-CRUSTED COD

SERVES 4

for a healthier take on fried fish

In North Carolina, we like to batter things up and deep-fry 'em—especially chicken, fish, and, yes, Twinkies—although in this book, we don't endorse the latter. Shalane's husband, Steve, grew up in Durham, NC, so after sharing the list of recipes with him, we weren't surprised when he commented that we should add something fried.

We started experimenting with frying fish but found that it made a spattering mess in our kitchens. We decided to try baking this cornmeal-crusted cod instead. Honest truth: The baked version turned out even more delicious.

A bonus: Instead of breadcrumbs, we use a stellar combo of cornmeal and almond meal in our battered cod, making this recipe gluten-free.

1 pound Pacific cod, skin and pin bones removed, cut into 4 fillets (ask your butcher to do this)

Fine sea salt

Freshly ground black pepper

⅓ cup fine cornmeal

1 egg

½ cup finely grated Parmesan cheese

½ cup almond meal

1 tablespoon minced fresh oregano leaves, dried well, or 1 teaspoon dried

1 tablespoon minced fresh thyme leaves, dried well, or 1 teaspoon dried

1 tablespoon extra-virgin olive oil

1. Rinse the fish and thoroughly pat it dry with paper towels. Sprinkle each fillet on all sides with salt and pepper.

2. Preheat the oven to 425°F. Place a wire rack on top of a baking sheet.

3. Line up three low-sided bowls on the counter. Place the cornmeal in the first bowl. Whisk the egg with 1 tablespoon water in the second bowl. In the third bowl, mix together the Parmesan, almond meal, oregano, and thyme.

4. Bread each fillet by dredging it in the cornmeal on all sides, then dipping it in the egg, then pressing it into the Parmesan mixture. Discard leftover breading mixtures.

5. Place the breaded fillets on top of the wire rack on the baking sheet. Drizzle lightly with the oil. Bake in the center of the oven until the fish flakes easily and is golden on top, 10 to 12 minutes. Use a metal spatula to remove from the rack and serve immediately.

PASTA PRIMAVERA WITH TEMPEH "SAUSAGE"

SERVES 4

for a dinner starring vegetables

1 package (8 ounces) tempeh

3 tablespoons extra-virgin olive oil

3 cloves garlic, minced

1 teaspoon dried oregano

1 teaspoon fennel seeds

¼ teaspoon red pepper flakes

1 large head broccoli (about 1 pound), cut into bite-size florets

2 cups sliced cremini or white button mushrooms

¼ teaspoon fine sea salt

½ cup dry white wine or low-sodium vegetable broth

1 recipe Simple Marinara Sauce (page 171) or 1 jar (26 ounces) marinara sauce

12 ounces dried pasta (gluten-free if sensitive)

½ cup grated Parmesan cheese (optional)

What runner doesn't love a big bowl of pasta? We know we certainly do. Even for those who are limiting their intake of refined carbohydrates, there can still be room to enjoy pasta. The thing is, most people have the ratio of noodles to sauce all wrong. When we serve pasta in our homes, we allow the sauce and vegetables to steal the limelight, not the pasta. This way, we're increasing our intake of the good stuff without overloading our system with processed grains. With sauce this good, we think you'll want to pile it high, too.

Never cooked tempeh before? Fear not. You need not be a veg-etarian or from Portlandia to enjoy this high-protein meat substi-tute. Those who dislike tofu or find it difficult to digest should give tempeh a try. Tempeh is made by fermenting whole soybeans, which means it's a lot less processed, easier to digest, and more flavorful than tofu. In this recipe, we simmer it in the sauce with garlic, oregano, and fennel—so flavorful your friends will probably mistake it for sausage.

1. In a food processor, pulse the tempeh until roughly ground.

2. In a large saucepan, warm the oil over medium heat. Add the garlic, oregano, fennel, and pepper flakes and cook, stirring continuously, until fragrant, 1 minute (be careful not to brown the garlic). Add the tempeh, broccoli, mushrooms, and salt and cook, stirring continuously, 5 to 6 minutes. Add the wine (or broth) and simmer just until it evaporates, about 2 minutes.

3. Add the marinara sauce and simmer for 10 to 15 minutes. Taste and add more salt and pepper flakes, if needed.

4. Meanwhile, cook the pasta according to package directions.

5. Divide the pasta into 4 bowls and top each with a heaping ladle of sauce and a sprinkle of Parmesan, if desired.

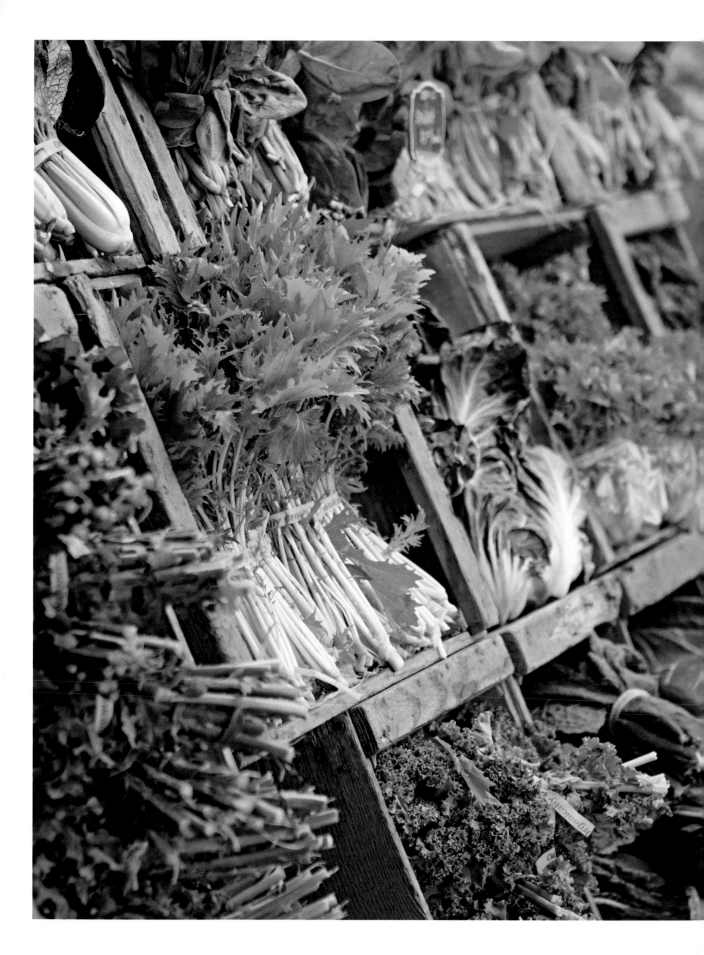

GIMME VEGGIES FRIED RICE

SERVES 4

for carbo-loading done right

2 tablespoons safflower oil or other high-heat oil

2 cloves garlic, minced

2 tablespoons finely chopped ginger

¼ teaspoon red pepper flakes

5 to 6 cups mixed chopped vegetables (carrots, celery, greens, bell pepper, peas, asparagus, etc.)

½ teaspoon fine sea salt

4 cups cooked short-grain brown rice, day old or chilled

2 tablespoons soy sauce (preferably tamari or shoyu)

2 eggs

1 teaspoon toasted sesame oil (optional)

3 scallions, thinly sliced (optional)

¼ cup chopped peanuts or cashews (optional)

Rice should be a go-to energy source in every runner's diet, especially rice dishes loaded with veggies and cooked full of satisfying umami flavor. Rice is an easily digestible source of complex carbohydrates and will fill you up without weighing you down.

This is the recipe we make at the end of the week when we peer into our fridge and see an odd assortment of veggies left over. It can be made with just about any veggie—our favorites include carrots, asparagus, and snow peas. If you want to add greens or mushrooms (yes, please!), add these quick-cooking veggies in the last couple of minutes since they give off a lot of moisture.

The key to great fried rice is to use short-grain brown rice because it maintains its satisfying chewy texture. For the best results, cook the rice the day before and take it straight from fridge to pan. This dish can also be cooked in a large skillet, but you will need to cut the recipe in half.

1. Heat a wok over high heat. Add 1 tablespoon of the oil and swirl to coat the bottom of the pan. Remove the wok from the heat and add the garlic, ginger, and pepper flakes. Cook briefly, stirring continuously, until fragrant, about 1 minute.

2. Return the wok to the heat and immediately add the mixed vegetables and salt. Cook, stirring occasionally, until the veggies are lightly browned and tender, 10 to 15 minutes. Transfer the veggies to a bowl.

3. Heat the remaining 1 tablespoon oil. Add the rice and soy sauce and cook, stirring occasionally, until lightly browned and toasty, about 3 minutes.

4. Reduce the heat to low and push the rice to one side. Crack the eggs on the other side and cook, stirring continuously, until scrambled. Stir the eggs into the rice, breaking up any clumps. Add the vegetables back to the wok and stir to combine.

5. Turn off the heat and stir in the sesame oil (if using). Taste and add more soy sauce, if needed. Serve immediately topped with the scallions and nuts (if using).

Make it a meal by adding in chopped chicken, shrimp, or tofu. Prior to cooking the vegetables, simply season your protein of choice with salt and pepper and sauté in a little oil. Set aside and toss back in just before serving.

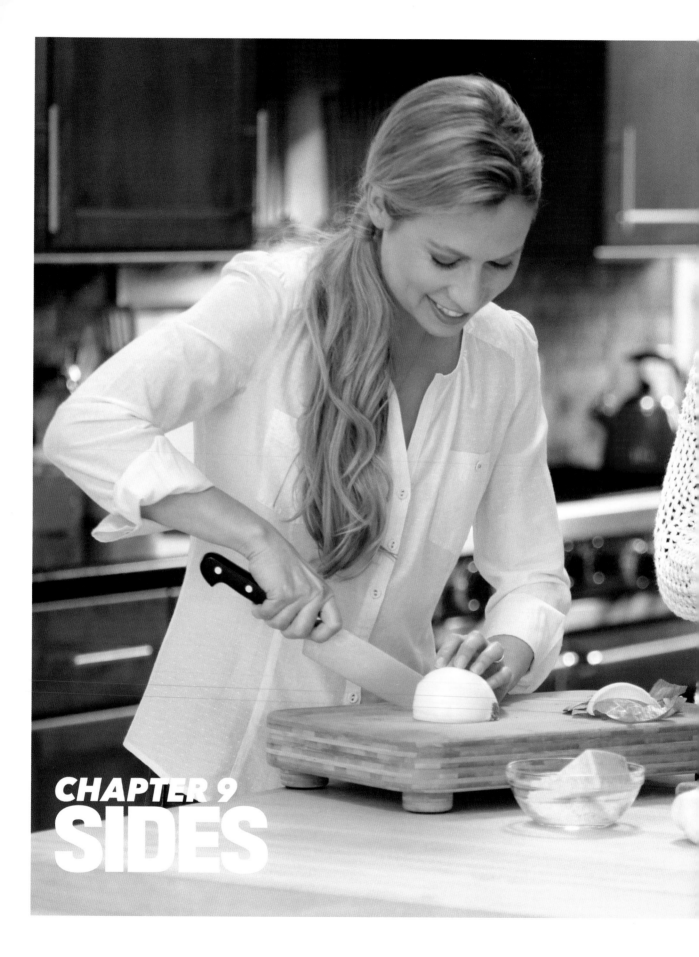

CHAPTER 9
SIDES

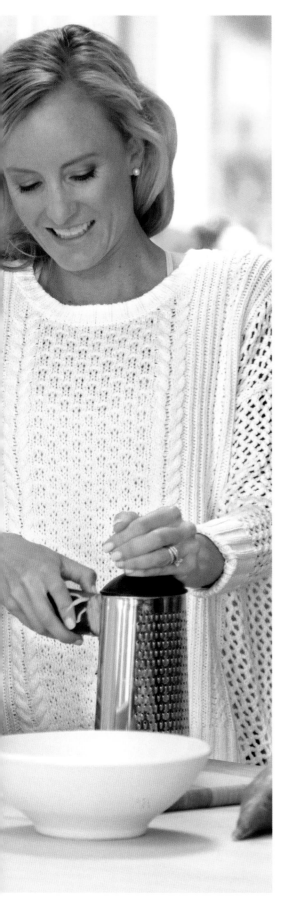

CAULIFLOWER COUSCOUS

MAKES 6 CUPS

for sneaking more veggies into your life

You don't need to be gluten-free to appreciate the incredible transformation cauliflower undergoes when pulsed finely and sautéed in a little olive oil. It takes on the taste and texture of couscous, only sweeter and fluffier.

Your significant other and any kiddos likely won't even notice when you swap this into your favorite couscous, bulgur, or rice recipes. We'll leave it up to you on how to best break the news to them that they just ate a bowlful of cauliflower and loved it!

1 large head cauliflower (1½ to 2 pounds)

2 tablespoons extra-virgin olive oil

1 teaspoon ground cumin

¼ teaspoon fine sea salt

¼ teaspoon freshly ground black pepper

1. Quarter the cauliflower head and cut off the individual florets.

2. In the work bowl of a food processor or professional blender, place the cauliflower florets, filling only halfway, and pulse several times until finely chopped. Transfer to a large bowl and continue with the remaining florets until all resemble couscous-size granules. If large pieces remain unchopped, remove them and process together at the end.

3. In a large skillet set over medium heat, warm the oil. Add the cauliflower, cumin, salt, and pepper and cook, stirring continuously, until the cauliflower is soft but still crisp, about 3 minutes.

4. Serve warm as a side dish or set aside to cool and toss into a salad. Pairs perfectly with our Moroccan Lentil Salad (page 96).

CHARRED CAULIFLOWER

SERVES 4

for satisfying a french fry craving

These cumin-spiked cauliflower bites give french fries a run for their money. Serve as an irresistible snack, a simple side dish, or a good-looking soup topper to replace soggy croutons. Our favorite way to devour these bites is on top of our Curry Lentil Soup (page 104).

Once you try our version, experiment with creating your own interpretation. Simply toss the cauliflower with any combination of spices or herbs that match the dish you are serving.

If your oven has a convection setting, use it here for crispier results in less time. Since convection runs hotter, you may want to turn the temperature down to 400°F and check the cauliflower after 20 minutes.

1 large head cauliflower, cut into similar-size florets (to ensure even cook time)

1 tablespoon extra-virgin olive oil

1 teaspoon ground cumin

½ teaspoon fine sea salt

1. Preheat the oven to 450°F.

2. Place the cauliflower florets on a large baking sheet and dry well with a paper towel. Add the oil, cumin, and salt and toss well to combine.

3. Spread out on the baking sheet and roast in the center of the oven until well browned and slightly charred, 25 to 30 minutes.

ROASTED BRUSSELS SPROUTS

SERVES 4

for a mighty veggie fix

These are better than buttered popcorn. We snack on them straight out of the oven. Keep it simple and let their natural sweetness shine. All you need is olive oil, salt, pepper, and high heat to bring out the best in this nutrient-packed cruciferous star.

2 pounds Brussels sprouts, stems trimmed, halved

2 tablespoon extra-virgin olive oil

½ teaspoon fine sea salt

¼ teaspoon freshly ground black pepper

1. Preheat the oven to 425°F. Line a rimmed baking sheet with parchment paper.

2. Place the Brussels sprouts on the baking sheet, toss them with the oil, salt, and pepper, and spread them out so they aren't touching.

3. Roast in the center of the oven, tossing once after 10 minutes, until tender in the center and charred on the outside, 20 to 25 minutes. Serve right out of the oven as a side dish.

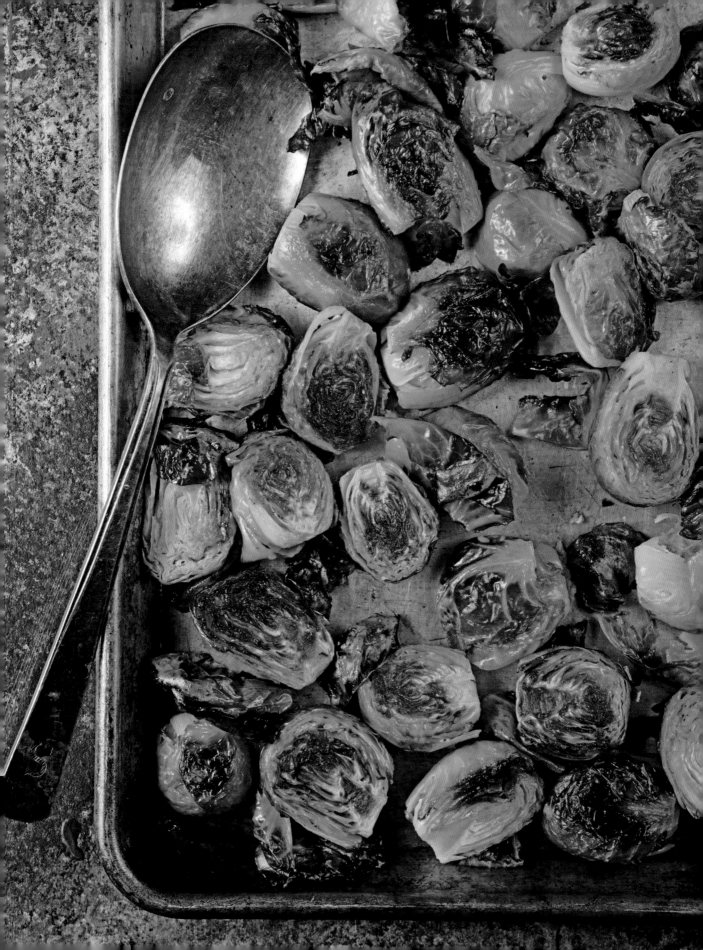

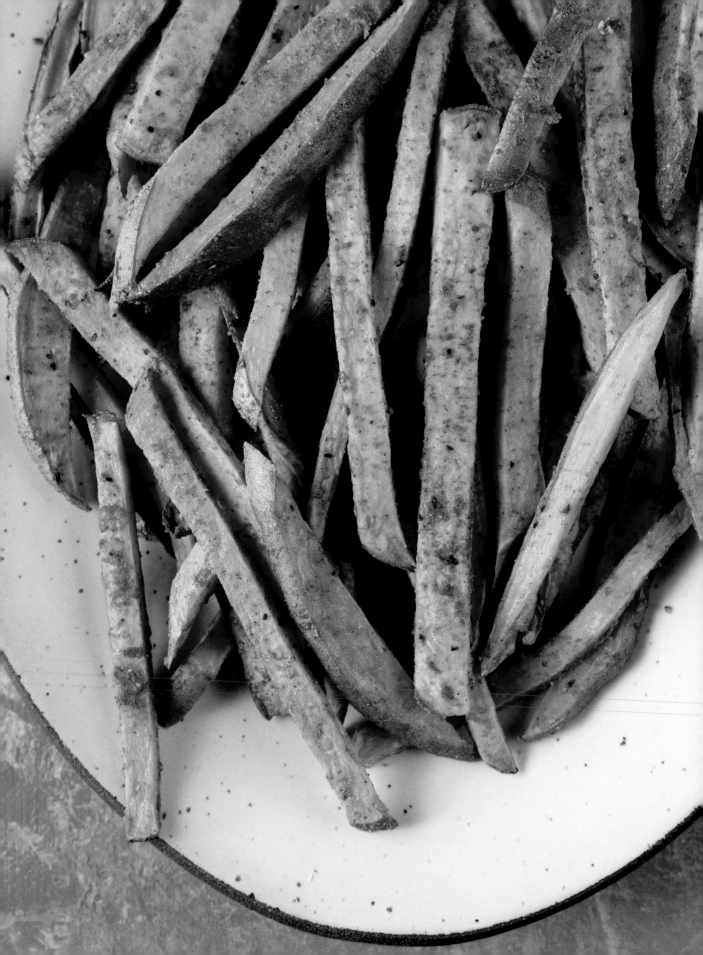

SWEET POTATO FRIES

SERVES 5

for whole foods carbo-loading

Mix up your roots. Try substituting parsnips for the yams. Simply increase the bake time by 5 to 10 minutes.

By now you're probably wondering just how many pounds of sweet potatoes we go through in a week. The answer is, a heckuva lot! We put sweet potatoes in everything from cookies (page 56) to salmon cakes (page 142) to lasagna (page 140) and more. We're madly in love with this deeply nourishing tuber. Orange-fleshed sweet potatoes (also called yams) are a highly digestible source of complex carbohydrates, providing balanced energy without the crash.

There's no need to peel these potatoes as there's awesome nutrition in the skin. Just give them a quick scrub. The addition of an egg white lends a crispy outer coating, but to make this recipe vegan, an extra tablespoon of olive oil can be used instead.

---

2 pounds (2 large or 3 medium) orange-fleshed sweet potatoes (yams)

1 egg white (save the yolk for breakfast), whisked

2 tablespoons extra-virgin olive oil

1½ tablespoons curry powder

¾ teaspoon fine sea salt

¼ teaspoon freshly ground black pepper

¼ teaspoon ground red pepper (optional, if you like spice)

1. Preheat the oven to 400°F. Line 2 baking sheets with parchment paper.

2. Cut the potatoes into sticks ¼ to ½ inch wide, as uniform in size as possible. Place the fries in a large mixing bowl and toss with the egg white and oil.

3. In a small bowl, mix together the curry powder, salt, black pepper, and red pepper (if using). Sprinkle the seasoning over the fries and toss until evenly combined.

4. Spread the fries on the baking sheets so they aren't touching one another (this ensures even cooking and crispiness). Place in the oven on the center and lower racks and bake for 20 minutes. Remove from the oven and use a spatula to flip the fries. Return to the oven and bake until the fries are browned on the outside and soft in the middle, about 10 minutes.

SPICY BLACK BEANS

MAKES 8 CUPS

for three meals in one

Got gas from beans? Adding kombu or epazote aids in the digestion of the gas-causing carbohydrates in beans. Learn more about seaweed on page 16.

Toss all the ingredients together in the pot of a slow cooker. Cook on high for 3 to 4 hours or low for 6 to 8 hours. Check partway through and add more water if the beans aren't fully submerged.

There are endless uses for a pot of well-seasoned black beans. In our homes, we like to make a big batch on Sundays and transform them into quick dinners all week long.

Start with the recipe below, and use the cooked beans in a variety of ways. Add ground meat and diced tomatoes to transform them into a flavorful chili. Add broth to turn them into black bean soup. Serve them on top of brown rice or a sweet potato with salsa, avocado, and cheese. Roll them into a burrito (like the Make-Ahead Breakfast Burrito on page 49), or turn them into a bean and cheese quesadilla for a late-night snack.

This recipe requires soaking the beans overnight prior to cooking.

2 tablespoons extra-virgin olive oil

1 yellow onion, chopped

2 carrots, diced

2 teaspoons fine sea salt

3 cloves garlic, smashed

1 pound dried black beans (2¼ cups), soaked in cold water overnight, drained, and rinsed

1 chipotle chile pepper in adobo (canned), chopped

3-inch-piece kombu or 1 sprig fresh epazote (or 1 tablespoon dried), optional (see tip opposite)

1 teaspoon ground cumin

1 bay leaf

1 tablespoon lime juice

1. Heat the oil in a large heavy-bottom pot over medium-high heat. Add the onion, carrots, and salt and cook, stirring occasionally, until softened, about 5 minutes. Add the garlic and cook for 1 minute.

2. Add the beans, chile pepper, kombu or epazote (if using), cumin, bay leaf, and just enough water to cover (about 4 to 5 cups). Bring to a boil. Cover, reduce the heat, and simmer for 1 to 2 hours, testing for doneness after 1 hour (beans should be creamy and easily mashed between two fingers).

3. To thicken the cooking liquid, smash a few beans with a fork and simmer uncovered until desired consistency is reached.

4. Prior to serving, add the lime juice, then taste and season with additional salt, if needed.

5. Serve warm, or allow to cool and store in gallon-size freezer bags in a flat layer, to make defrosting easier.

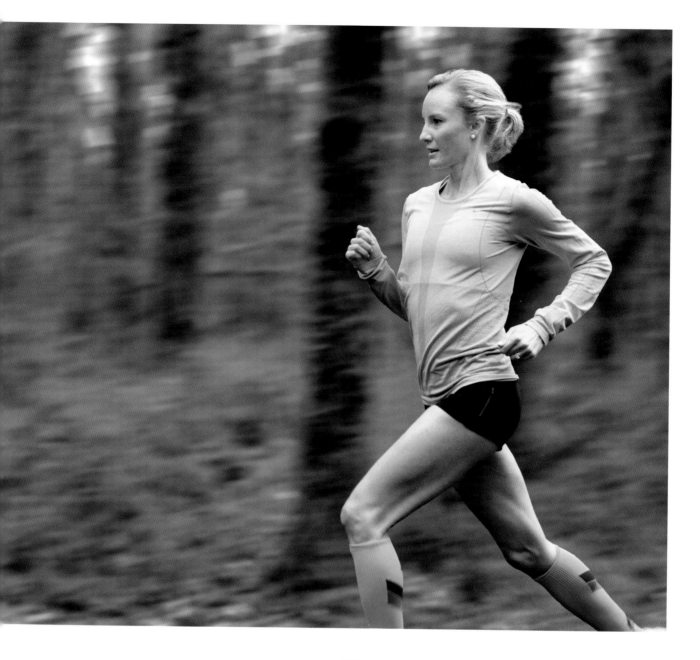

TIP

Beans absorb varying amounts of water, depending on
how long they have been in storage and how long
they soak prior to cooking. To prevent burning, keep an eye
on your beans, and if they aren't fully submerged in water,
add another cup partway through cooking.

TIP

Freeze leftover chipotle chile peppers in a single layer to use
for future recipes like Chipotle Hummus (page 70).

GARLICKY GREENS

SERVES 4

for bone-building nourishment

Step aside, kale! As an ode to our Carolina days, we had to include a recipe for collard greens. Collards are simply incredible. They're so nutrient-rich that once we started eating them, we found ourselves craving them for breakfast. Luckily the leftovers are delicious topped with a fried egg.

Despite our Southern roots, we like our greens sautéed in a little oil with plenty of garlic, a few spices, and a squeeze of lemon juice. In our recipe, no ham hock or long simmer in stock is needed to make them burst with flavor. We prefer our collards cooked lightly to maintain their vibrant color and delicious chewy texture.

Collard greens are rich in too many vitamins and minerals to list out here. Look 'em up. You'll be impressed.

---

2 bunches collard greens, stems removed

2 tablespoons virgin coconut oil or extra-virgin olive oil

6 cloves garlic, minced

1 teaspoon cumin seeds

1 teaspoon fennel seeds

½ teaspoon red pepper flakes (optional, if you like spice)

½ teaspoon fine sea salt

1 tablespoon lemon juice

1. Stack the collard leaves, roll them together lengthwise, and cut into ½-inch ribbons.

2. Heat the oil in a large skillet with a lid over medium heat. Add the garlic, cumin, fennel, and pepper flakes (if using) and cook briefly, stirring continuously, until fragrant (be careful not to brown the garlic).

3. Add the greens and salt and cook, stirring frequently, until wilted, about 3 minutes.

4. Turn the heat to low, cover, and cook until tender, about 3 minutes.

5. Turn off the heat, stir in the lemon juice, taste, and season with additional salt, if needed.

MASHED YAMS WITH SAGE BROWN BUTTER

SERVES 6

for mixing up tradition

🕐 This dish can be prepared 1 to 2 days in advance. Simply skip baking the mixture and store covered in the fridge. Take out of the fridge 1 hour prior to baking to bring it up to room temperature, then follow the last step below.

Holiday dinners require plenty of side dishes. In our opinion, the sides are more important (and more fun to cook!) than the main dish. The turkey is simply a vehicle for scooping up all those luscious sides.

But many of the traditional sides we grew up eating are shockingly high in processed ingredients—like the canned fried onions and condensed cream of mushroom soup in Mom's green bean casserole and the canned yams, brown sugar, and marshmallows in her candied yams (sorry, Mom!). But instead of tossing these traditions out the window, we've evolved these recipes to make use of ingredients we can feel good about serving to our families.

Our mashed yams are always a devoured favorite at Thanksgiving. The natural sweetness in the yams contrasts harmoniously with the savory toppings.

3½ to 4 pounds orange-fleshed sweet potatoes (yams)

1 recipe Sage Brown Butter (page 172)

½ cup whole milk

½ teaspoon fine sea salt

¼ teaspoon freshly ground black pepper

Pinch of ground nutmeg (optional)

½ cup grated Parmesan cheese

¼ cup raw pumpkin seeds

1. Preheat the oven to 400°F.

2. Wrap the sweet potatoes individually in foil and bake in the center of the oven until very soft, 55 to 60 minutes. Allow them to cool enough to handle, then remove the skin, place in a large mixing bowl, and use a fork to mash until smooth.

3. Add the butter, milk, salt, pepper, and nutmeg (if using) and mix until combined. Taste and add a little more salt, if needed.

4. Reduce the oven temperature to 350°F. Transfer the mixture to an 8 x 8-inch baking dish. Top with the cheese and pumpkin seeds.

5. Bake for 20 to 25 minutes, or until the cheese is melted and the potatoes are warm in the center, 20 to 25 minutes.

CHAPTER 10
SAUCES AND DRESSINGS

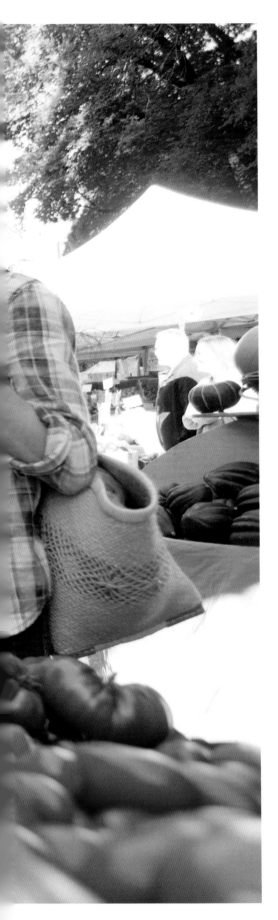

LEMON MISO DRESSING

MAKES ABOUT 1 CUP

for dressing up in style

This is our signature dressing. 'Nuff said. Make it tonight and you won't be disappointed.

This dressing has a special affinity for our Kale-Radicchio Salad with Farro (page 80). It's our go-to salad that we take to just about every baby shower, potluck dinner, and picnic. We'll keep making it because our friends keep requesting it—and we're starting to wonder if they're inviting us or our salad over!

½ cup extra-virgin olive oil

⅓ cup lemon juice

2 or 3 cloves garlic, minced

2 teaspoons miso paste (preferably mellow white)

½ teaspoon fine sea salt

¼ teaspoon freshly ground black pepper

1. Combine the oil, lemon juice, garlic, miso, salt, and pepper in a glass jar with a lid. Use a fork to stir in the miso, then shake vigorously to emulsify.

2. Pour generously over your favorite grain salad.

3. This dressing will keep in the fridge for up to 1 week. If the oil solidifies, briefly microwave on low until melted.

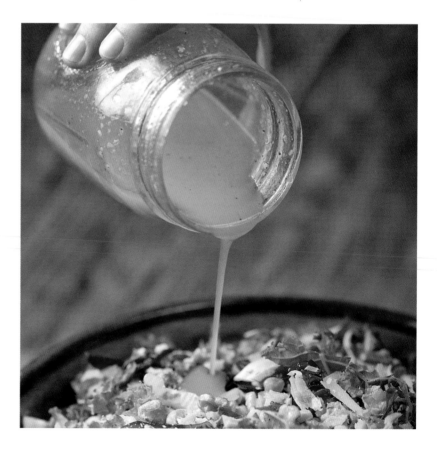

BASIC BALSAMIC VINAIGRETTE

MAKES ⅔ CUP

for versatility

For an unbeatable easy summer dinner, pair this vinaigrette with Strawberry-Arugula Kamut Salad (page 81).

Elyse hasn't bought bottled salad dressing in 10 years—not since she met her French-American husband, Andy, and quickly learned that homemade salad dressing is about the easiest thing to whip together. A flawless salad dressing really only needs three ingredients: oil, vinegar, and emulsifier (Dijon in this case). Compare that to the ingredient label on your store-bought dressing and you'll be convinced to make your own.

For best results, use real balsamic vinegar and high-quality olive oil. Check the label when buying balsamic vinegar. Many of the less expensive brands are simply wine vinegars with coloring (caramel color) and sweeteners. True balsamic vinegar is expensive, but the deep oaky flavor makes it worth its hefty price tag.

Elyse converted Shalane into a salad dressing-making goddess, and now not a week goes by that Shalane isn't shaking up a batch of this versatile vinaigrette.

⅓ cup extra-virgin olive oil

¼ cup balsamic vinegar

1 heaping tablespoon Dijon mustard

1. Combine the oil, vinegar, and mustard in a glass jar with a lid. Shake vigorously until emulsified.

2. This dressing will keep in the fridge for up to 1 month (if it doesn't have fresh herbs, shallots, or garlic added). If the oil solidifies, briefly microwave on low until melted.

TIP

Mix it up by adding minced garlic or shallots and fresh herbs.

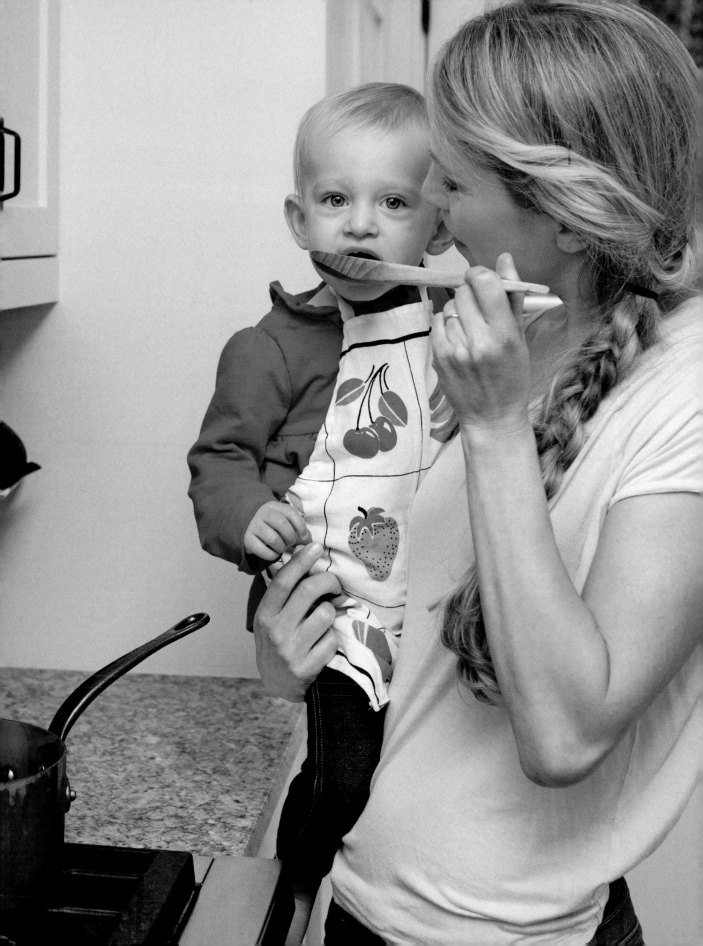

SIMPLE MARINARA SAUCE

MAKES 2 QUARTS

for endless options

Make a double batch in a large pot and freeze half—you'll be one step ahead of the game. See the recipe ideas at right.

This basic but mighty marinara sauce makes a terrific base for endless dishes. It's a jumping-off point for our Marathon Lasagna (page 140), Pasta Primavera with Tempeh "Sausage" (page 151), and High-Altitude Bison Meatballs (page 120). It's also superb smothered on top of our Millet Pizza Pies (page 133) with any assortment of your favorite pizza toppings.

If you're serving it straight up without adding seasoned ground meat, we recommend adding a few pinches of red pepper flakes to heat up the flavor.

---

3 tablespoons extra-virgin olive oil

2 large carrots, peeled and finely chopped

1 large yellow onion, finely chopped

3 cloves garlic, minced

1 teaspoon fine sea salt

2 cans (28 ounces each) whole or diced tomatoes

1 tablespoon minced fresh oregano or 2 teaspoons dried

½ teaspoon freshly ground black pepper

¼ to ½ teaspoon red pepper flakes (optional, if you like spice)

Handful of fresh basil leaves, chopped (optional)

1. Heat the oil in a large saucepan over medium heat. Add the carrots, onion, garlic, and salt and cook, stirring frequently, until the onions are soft but not brown, about 8 minutes.

2. Add the tomatoes (along with their juices), oregano, black pepper, and pepper flakes (if using). If the tomatoes are whole, break them up into small pieces with a wooden spoon. Bring to a simmer and cook uncovered, until the sauce thickens, stirring occasionally, at least 30 minutes or up to 1 hour 30 minutes for a thicker, richer sauce.

3. Leave the sauce chunky or blend with an immersion (stick) blender until smooth. Taste and add more salt and pepper, if needed.

4. Just before serving, stir in the basil (if using).

TIP

Some brands of canned tomatoes are less sweet than others. If your sauce tastes too acidic, add 1 tablespoon coconut sugar or other granulated sugar.

SAGE BROWN BUTTER

SERVES 4

for a 5-minute sauce

We classify butter as a super-awesome food. Learn why on page 17.

As long as you don't walk away from the stove, this is about the easiest (and most outrageously delicious) sauce you can whip together to toss with any assortment of vegetables and pasta. After the butter melts, the tiny milk protein particles will separate out and begin to turn brown. If it looks like sand in your pan, fear not, this is a good thing; keep going until the particles turn deep brown and the butter smells toasty.

We love this nutty, caramelized sauce drizzled on baked fish, but our all-time favorite pairings are Penne with Roasted Butternut Squash (page 135) or Mashed Yams (page 165).

4 tablespoons unsalted butter

¼ cup finely chopped fresh sage leaves

Fine sea salt

Freshly ground black pepper

1. In a large saucepan or skillet over medium heat, melt the butter and continue cooking, stirring occasionally, until the butter turns golden brown with tiny brown flecks, 4 to 5 minutes.

2. Remove the pan from the heat, slowly add the sage leaves, and stir. Add salt and pepper to taste.

APPLE CIDER VINAIGRETTE

MAKES ½ CUP

for brightening any salad

Apple cider vinegar is inexpensive and crazy good for you. It's high in minerals, can help your body maintain healthy pH levels, and is rich in digestion-enhancing enzymes. We're so hooked on making salad dressings out of it that we're giving you three variations to try.

All three variations (even the creamy version) are vegan-friendly. When buying apple cider vinegar, the uglier the better. If it's clear instead of murky, the "mother" (enzymes and good bacteria) has been filtered out.

⅓ cup extra-virgin olive oil

¼ cup apple cider vinegar

1 tablespoon Dijon mustard

½ shallot, minced

¼ teaspoon fine sea salt

¼ teaspoon freshly ground black pepper

1. Combine the oil, vinegar, mustard, shallot, salt, and pepper in a glass jar with a lid. Shake vigorously until emulsified.

2. This basic vinaigrette pairs happily with any refreshing salad. We are partial to pouring it generously over our Green Apple-Fennel Salad with Hazelnuts (page 88).

3. This dressing will keep in the fridge for up to 1 week. If the oil solidifies, briefly microwave on low until melted.

CREAMY APPLE CIDER VINAIGRETTE

Add 2 tablespoons tahini to the above. The creamy variation pairs perfectly with our Wild West Rice Salad (page 90).

MAPLE-DIJON APPLE CIDER VINAIGRETTE

Add 2 teaspoons maple syrup to the basic recipe. This sweet variation goes superbly with lentil salads. Try it on our Moroccan Lentil Salad with Cauliflower Couscous (page 96).

CILANTRO-LIME CASHEW SAUCE

MAKES 1½ CUPS

for easy weeknight dinners

We're the sauce-loving types. Simple dishes can be transformed into whoa-nelly magic with the right drizzle. But sauces are high in fat, which is bad, right? Think again, my friend. Homemade sauces like ours are made with fueling fats. For athletes, a diet rich in good fats is paramount to health and happiness (read our full spiel on fats on page 6).

This creamy sauce is made with cashews instead of milk, making it a coveted sauce for those avoiding dairy. And it just might make your household fight over the bowl of veggies.

1 cup unroasted cashews

¾ cup boiling water

1 cup loosely packed cilantro leaves

¼ cup lime juice (2 or 3 limes)

2 cloves garlic

1 tablespoon extra-virgin olive oil

1 teaspoon miso paste (preferably white, see page 19)

¾ teaspoon fine sea salt

1. Soak the cashews in the boiling water for 30 minutes (or overnight, covered and refrigerated). Place the cashews, the soaking water, cilantro, lime juice, garlic, oil, miso, and salt in a high-speed blender or food processor and blend until completely smooth.

2. Serve drizzled on top of your favorite stir-fried or roasted veggies and rice.

3. Store in an airtight container in the fridge for up to 5 days. If the sauce thickens, thin with a tablespoon or two of water.

RUNNER'S HIGH PEANUT SAUCE

MAKES 2⅓ CUPS

for postrun nourishment

Transfer any leftover sauce to a jar with a tight-fitting lid and refrigerate for up to 5 days. Or freeze individual portions in a silicone muffin tray and then transfer to a gallon-size freezer bag.

Fill your rice bowl with a full rainbow of vegetables to max out on disease-fighting phytonutrients.

When we began recipe development, one of Shalane's first requests was for an alluring sauce to drizzle on top of seasonal veggies and rice for an easy postrun meal. She knew that store-bought sauces, although really convenient, are often loaded with sugar, cheap oils, and preservatives.

And so our Runner's High Peanut Sauce was born. This is a phenomenal sauce so good you'll be tempted to drink the leftovers—that is, if there are any. We recommend making a double batch so you can freeze leftovers in individual serving sizes for quick meals after a hard workout. (It freezes superbly.) While training with the Bowerman Track Club at high altitude in Park City, Utah, Shalane made a quadruple batch of this sauce to share with her teammates.

Yes, it's slightly more work than opening a jar, but trust us, it's well worth the effort. This sauce pairs heavenly with sautéed vegetables and brown rice or our Soba Noodle Salad (page 87).

---

1 tablespoon virgin coconut oil or extra-virgin olive oil

1 yellow onion, diced

½ teaspoon fine sea salt

3 cloves garlic, minced

1 can (13½ ounces) unsweetened coconut milk (preferably full-fat)

½ cup unsalted creamy peanut butter (100% peanuts)

1 tablespoon soy sauce (preferably shoyu or tamari)

1 tablespoon coconut sugar or other granulated sugar

½ to 1 teaspoon red pepper flakes, depending on spice preference

1 tablespoon lime juice (about ½ lime)

¼ cup chopped peanuts

1. In a medium saucepan over medium-high heat, warm the oil. Add the onion and salt and cook, stirring occasionally, until soft but not brown, about 5 minutes. Add the garlic and cook, stirring frequently, for 1 minute.

2. Add the coconut milk, peanut butter, soy sauce, sugar, and pepper flakes. Bring to a simmer and whisk until the peanut butter melts. Reduce the heat to low and simmer, uncovered, stirring occasionally, until the sauce thickens and the flavors meld, about 10 minutes. Remove the pan from the heat and stir in the lime juice.

3. Using an immersion (stick) blender, if you have one, blend the sauce until smooth. Alternatively, transfer the sauce to the container of a blender and process until the sauce is smooth.

4. To serve, fill a bowl with cooked brown rice, add your favorite sautéed veggies, top generously with the sauce, and garnish with the peanuts.

MIGHTY MARINADE

MAKES ABOUT 1 CUP

for infusing flavor

We call this our Mighty Marinade because it doesn't rely on sugar or artificial ingredients to infuse your meat or veggies with mighty good flavor. And it works effortlessly on chicken, steak, pork chops, fish, veggies, or tempeh.

New to grilling? Here's our best advice: Don't micromanage the grill. While it's tempting to constantly peek at your food to check that it hasn't gone up in flames, it's best to resist opening the lid as much as possible. Every time you lift the cover, the temperature drops drastically. When cooking on a grill, the surrounding indirect heat is as important as the direct heat to ensure the food cooks through instead of just searing it on the outside. You also want to resist the urge to flip the meat and vegetables back and forth. Cooking once per side will give you the best results. Bring a timer outside with you and set it for the recommended cook time.

This recipe makes enough marinade for 2 pounds of meat or veggies. The marinade times vary based on what you're grilling, so for the best results consult our handy chart opposite.

2 tablespoons extra-virgin olive oil

¼ cup lime juice (1 to 2 limes), plus half a lime to squeeze over meat during grilling

¼ cup soy sauce (preferably shoyu or tamari)

3 cloves garlic, smashed

2-inch knob fresh ginger, grated, or 1 teaspoon ground

2 tablespoons honey

1. In a gallon-size freezer bag, combine the oil, lime juice, soy sauce, garlic, ginger, and honey. Add the meat or veggies, seal the bag, and shake well to combine.

2. Place the bag in the fridge and allow the meat or veggies to marinate for the time listed opposite.

3. Bring the meat or veggies to room temperature by removing the bag from the fridge 30 minutes prior to grilling. Preheat the grill to medium-high and cook according to the chart opposite.

4. When placing meat on the grill, first shake off any excess marinade, then stand back to avoid the flare-up. To brighten the flavor, halfway through cooking squeeze a little lime juice over top of the meat.

Grill Chart

	MARINATE TIME	COOK TIME
Boneless, skinless chicken	4 to 24 hours	4 to 6 minutes per side
Pork chops	4 to 24 hours	3 to 4 minutes per side
Skin-on chicken	12 to 24 hours	8 to 10 minutes per side
Steak	12 to 24 hours	3 to 6 minutes per side depending on thickness and rareness preference
Fish	30 minutes	5 minutes per side for every inch thickness
Tempeh	4 to 24 hours	5 minutes per side
Veggies	30 minutes	Delicate veggies about 5 minutes, hearty veggies about 10 minutes, rotating frequently

AVOCADO CREAM

SERVES 4

for a nondairy creamy kick

If we were stranded on an island, we're pretty sure we could survive just fine as long as we had an avocado tree. Avocados are an incredible, vitamin-rich fruit loaded with energy-giving fats. Walk into our kitchens any day of the week and you'll see avocados ripening on our counters.

For our running friends who are lactose intolerant or follow a vegan diet, we wanted to create a nondairy alternative to take Shalane's Breakfast-Meets-Dinner Bowl (page 128), or any rice bowl for that matter, over the top. We're so in love with the results that we now also put our Avocado Cream on our Make-Ahead Breakfast Burritos (page 49), Greek Bison Burgers (page 138), Pita Chips with Oregano and Sea Salt (page 74), and baked fish.

For a fiery cream, include the seeds of the jalapeño. For a mild version, leave the seeds out.

---

2 small or 1 large ripe avocado, halved

1 small or ½ large jalapeño chile pepper, stem removed, quartered (wear plastic gloves when handling)

2 teaspoons lime juice

1 tablespoon extra-virgin olive oil

¼ teaspoon fine sea salt

1. Scoop the meat from the avocado and place in a food processor with the chile pepper, lime juice, oil, and salt. Process until smooth and transfer to a bowl.

2. Or prepare by hand by mashing the avocado with a fork until smooth in a medium bowl. Finely chop the chile pepper and add to the bowl along with the lime juice, oil, and salt and stir to combine.

3. Cover the bowl tightly with plastic wrap and refrigerate until ready to use. Store any leftovers in an airtight container in the fridge for up to 1 day.

DULSE MINERAL SALT

MAKES ½ CUP

for a mighty mineral boost

Shake up your condiments! Here's a recipe for a satisfying salt made with seaweed. We keep small mason jars of this on our kitchen tables alongside the salt and pepper for when we need a mighty mineral boost. Seaweed is a superfood for athletes as it's loaded with B_{12} (superb for vegans and vegetarians) and iron. It adds a nice salty crunch to rice bowls, stir-fries, salads, soups, roasted veggies, baked potatoes, and fish.

For a mineral-rich, addicting snack, sprinkle generously on half an avocado and devour with a spoon. Seaweed is extremely high in iodine (great for those with an underactive thyroid) but should not be consumed in large quantities (especially if you have an overactive thyroid).

Dulse can be found at most natural foods stores or ordered online (see Resources on page 220).

---

3 tablespoons sesame seeds

1 ounce dried dulse (whole, not flakes or granules; see seaweed on page 16 to learn more)

1 teaspoon safflower oil or other neutral high-heat oil

¼ teaspoon fine sea salt

1. Heat a dry cast-iron skillet over medium heat. Add the seeds and toast until fragrant, stirring frequently, about 5 minutes (being careful not to let them brown). Set the seeds aside to cool.

2. Separate the clumps of dulse into smaller pieces and check for any debris (you might find the remains of a seashell!). Warm the oil in the same skillet over medium heat. Add the dulse and salt and toast until crispy (the color will lighten), stirring frequently, about 5 minutes. Watch it carefully to avoid burning.

3. Transfer the dulse to a mortar and use a pestle to crush into small flakes. Alternatively, transfer the dulse to a regular bowl, allow it to cool, and crumble it by hand. If any pieces are too moist to crumble, return them to the skillet and toast for an additional minute.

4. Add the sesame seeds and stir to combine. Transfer to a small glass jar with a lid.

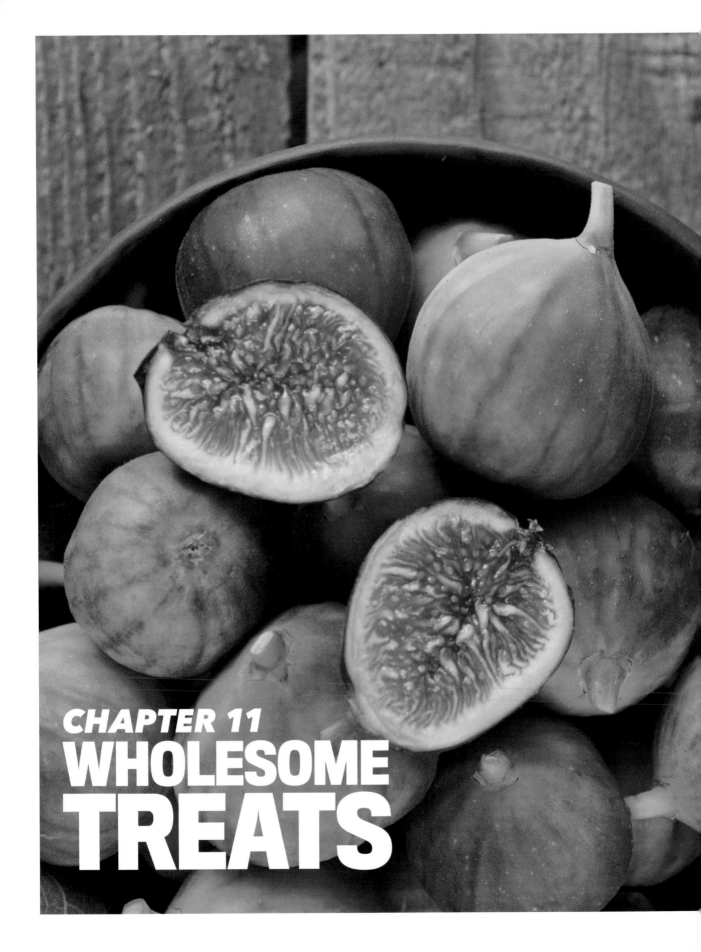

CHAPTER 11
WHOLESOME
TREATS

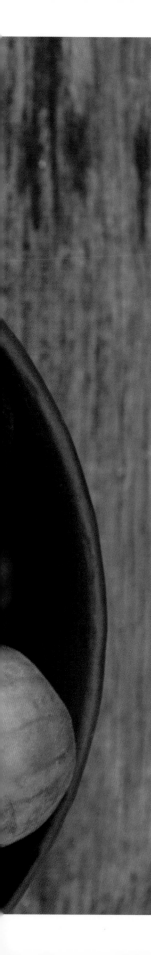

GINGER-MOLASSES QUICK BREAD

MAKES 1 LOAF

for an iron-pumping loaf

1½ cups dark rye flour or whole wheat or spelt flour

1-inch knob fresh ginger, peeled and grated, or 1 teaspoon ground

½ teaspoon ground cinnamon

½ teaspoon fine sea salt

2 teaspoons baking powder

1 teaspoon baking soda

1 egg

1 cup whole milk yogurt

½ cup molasses

4 tablespoons unsalted butter, melted

¼ cup golden raisins

1 teaspoon orange zest (optional)

Baking bread is rewarding, especially when it's a sweetly spiced loaf that fills your entire home with aromas reminiscent of the holidays. This recipe is adapted from a favorite in the 1975 edition of *Joy of Cooking*. The current authors of *Joy of Cooking*, Megan Scott and John Becker, shared this recipe with us and we adapted it to a runner's needs (and sweet cravings).

Instead of refined sugar and nutrient-stripped wheat flour, we've swapped in molasses and rye flour. Molasses is crazy high in iron, potassium, and calcium—a sweet bonus. And the rye flour lends a robust nutty flavor and rich nutrient-profile. (Because it is difficult to separate the germ and bran from the endosperm of rye, rye flour has more nutrients than refined wheat flour.)

Not all breads require hours of kneading to bake into wholesome perfection. The thing we love about quick breads is they're just that—quick. Whisk together the dry ingredients, whisk together the wet ingredients, combine, pour into a loaf pan and you're done. No sweat, my friend.

Serve with a mugful of our Runner's Recovery Iced Tea (page 36) and you'll be good to go.

1. Preheat the oven to 350° F. Grease an 8½ x 4½-inch loaf pan with butter.

2. In a medium bowl, whisk together the flour, ginger, cinnamon, salt, baking powder, and baking soda.

3. In a separate small bowl, whisk together the egg, yogurt, molasses, butter, raisins, and orange zest (if using). Add to the dry ingredients and stir just enough to bring the batter together. Do not overmix. The batter will be very thick.

4. Pour into the loaf pan and bake until a butter knife inserted into the center comes out clean, 40 to 45 minutes.

5. Cool in the pan for 10 minutes, then transfer the loaf to a wire rack and allow to cool completely prior to slicing.

SPELT BANANA BREAD

MAKES 1 LOAF

for wholesome energy

For banana bread muffins, line a muffin pan with 12 paper muffin cups. Fill each cup with batter, then bake until golden, 20 to 25 minutes.

We runners love our bananas—and for good reason. Bananas are a highly digestible source of energy that can quickly replenish depleted glycogen levels in our hardworking muscles. They're also a fantastic natural source of electrolytes, including potassium and magnesium.

But before you go chowing down on Mom's banana bread, take a peek at the list of ingredients. Most banana breads are loaded with sugar and cheap vegetable oils. We took her recipe and gave it a makeover by sneaking in performance-boosting ingredients such as whole grain spelt flour and real butter. The key to achieving sweet perfection with a lot less sugar is to use very, very ripe bananas.

Now go put those long-forgotten brown-speckled bananas to good use.

1½ cups spelt flour

1 teaspoon ground cinnamon

1 teaspoon baking soda

½ teaspoon fine sea salt

1 stick (½ cup) unsalted butter, at room temperature

¼ cup coconut sugar or other granulated sugar

2 eggs

1½ cups mashed banana (3 or 4 very ripe, brown-speckled bananas)

1 teaspoon vanilla extract

½ cup chopped toasted walnuts (optional)

½ cup date pieces or golden raisins (optional)

1. Preheat the oven to 350°F. Grease a 8½ x 4½-inch loaf pan with butter.

2. In a large mixing bowl, combine the flour, cinnamon, baking soda, and salt.

3. In a separate mixing bowl, use a handheld mixer or stand mixer to beat together the butter and sugar on low just until combined. Add the eggs and continue to beat for 1 minute. Add the bananas and vanilla and beat just until combined.

4. Pour the wet ingredients over the dry ingredients and stir just until combined. Fold in the walnuts and dates or raisins (if using).

5. Pour into the loaf pan and shake the pan to spread the batter evenly. Bake in the center of the oven until the top is golden brown and a knife inserted in the center comes out clean, 50 to 60 minutes.

6. Transfer the pan to a wire rack and cool for 15 minutes. Run a knife around the edges to loosen and carefully flip to remove the loaf. Cool completely on the wire rack prior to slicing.

FLOURLESS ALMOND TORTE

SERVES 12

for the love of real cake

This rustic, low-maintenance cake is a cinch to prep and can be served endless ways. In summer, try it topped with fresh berries and whipped cream. In fall, serve it with warm Sautéed Pears (page 186) and vanilla ice cream.

To achieve a moist, delicate cake, use almond flour, which is made from blanched, skinless almonds, instead of almond meal. The leftovers are hearty enough—and wholesome enough—to devour for breakfast (you have our full permission).

Unsalted butter at room temperature

6 eggs

1 cup maple syrup

¼ cup extra-virgin olive oil

2 teaspoons almond extract

1 tablespoon lemon zest (zest of 2 large lemons)

½ teaspoon fine sea salt

5 cups almond flour (not almond meal)

1 cup raw sliced almonds

1. Preheat the oven to 350°F. Grease a 9-inch springform (removable sides) cake pan with the butter.

2. In a large mixing bowl, whisk together the eggs, maple syrup, oil, almond extract, lemon zest, and salt. Add the almond flour and stir until thoroughly combined.

3. Pour the batter into the cake pan and sprinkle the sliced almonds over top. Bake in the center of the oven until a toothpick inserted in the center comes out clean, 40 to 45 minutes.

4. Cool the cake in the pan on a wire rack. Carefully slide a thin knife around the edges of the cake and remove the pan's sides. Slide the knife underneath the cake to loosen and transfer it to a serving dish. Cut it into 12 slices.

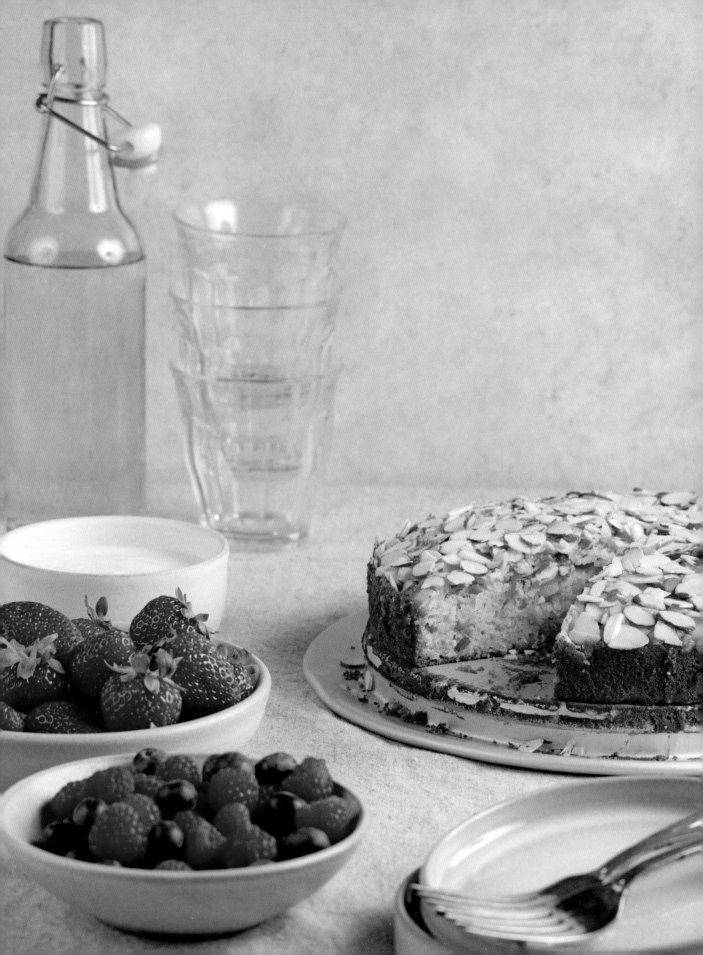

SAUTÉED PEARS

SERVES 4

for the ultimate sundae

When fresh berries aren't in season, fragrant sautéed pears are delicious spooned over a slice of our unforgettable Flourless Almond Torte (page 184) or vanilla ice cream.

1 tablespoon virgin coconut oil or unsalted butter

2 ripe pears (firm variety like Anjou or Bosc), peeled and sliced ½-inch thick

1 teaspoon ground cinnamon

Pinch of fine sea salt

1 tablespoon maple syrup

1 teaspoon lemon juice

1. Heat the oil or butter in a small skillet over medium heat. Add the pears, cinnamon, and salt and cook, stirring frequently, until the pears soften and release juices, about 5 minutes.

2. Remove the pan from the heat and stir in the maple syrup and lemon juice. Serve warm.

DOUBLE CHOCOLATE TEFF COOKIES

MAKES 18 COOKIES

for satisfying a serious chocolate craving

Here's a little secret: Shalane has a serious hankering for sweet treats, especially chocolate. While crafting the list of recipes for this book, Elyse kept receiving one-line e-mails from Shalane requesting more goodies. Luckily for Shalane, Elyse considers dark chocolate a health food, especially chocolatey treats that are free of refined sugars and made with whole grains (like these bad boys).

These gluten-free cookies are made with the nutritional powerhouse that is teff, the whole grain of choice among Ethiopian runners (learn more about teff on page 14). Teff has a nutty, chocolatey aroma that really comes to life when paired with cocoa powder.

This is the adored treat that Shalane made most frequently for her fellow teammates while training at 7,000 feet in Park City, Utah. For best results, we recommend allowing the batter to rest overnight in the fridge prior to baking. This gives the whole grain flour the chance to soften for a more tender cookie.

¾ cup teff flour (make sure the bag says "flour")

½ cup almond flour or almond meal

⅓ cup semisweet chocolate chips

¼ cup unsweetened cocoa powder

1 teaspoon baking powder

¼ teaspoon baking soda

¼ teaspoon fine sea salt

½ cup pure maple syrup

⅓ cup coconut oil, melted

1 teaspoon vanilla extract

1. In a large bowl, whisk together the teff flour, almond flour, chocolate chips, cocoa powder, baking powder, baking soda, and salt.

2. Add the maple syrup, oil, and vanilla and stir just until combined. For a more tender cookie, cover the batter and refrigerate overnight prior to baking.

3. Preheat the oven to 350°F. Line a baking sheet with parchment paper.

4. Drop the batter by heaping tablespoons 1 inch apart on the baking sheet.

5. Bake in the center of the oven until the bottoms are lightly browned, 12 minutes. Let the cookies cool for 5 minutes, then transfer to a rack to cool completely.

STONE FRUIT MINI PIES WITH PRESSED NUT CRUST

MAKES 6 MINI PIES OR 9 MUFFIN-SIZE PIES

for summer bliss

CRUST

1½ cups raw pecans or walnuts

1 cup rolled oats (gluten-free if sensitive)

8 Deglet dates, pitted

1 teaspoon ground cinnamon

¼ teaspoon fine sea salt

1 egg

1 teaspoon vanilla extract

FILLING

1½ pounds ripe stone fruit (about 3 peaches or 4 plums or apricots), chopped into ½-inch pieces

2 tablespoons coconut sugar or other granulated sugar

1 tablespoon lemon juice

1 tablespoon tapioca starch or cornstarch

½ teaspoon ground cinnamon

⅛ teaspoon ground cardamom or nutmeg (optional)

These adorable pies beg you to slow down, pour a cup of coffee or tea, and savor every bite. Because we couldn't decide which stone fruit we liked best (all three were winners!), we leave it up to you to fill your pies with any assortment of them. (Come wintertime, sub in ripe pears!)

These nourishing pies are made with nothing but the best. Because they're basically oats, nuts, and fruit, this is a dessert you're allowed to devour before noon. Serve them with a scoop of whole milk plain yogurt and you've got a complete breakfast.

1. *To make the crust:* Preheat the oven to 350°F. Butter 6 mini-pie pans (as pictured) or 9 cups of a muffin pan.

2. In a food processor, combine the nuts, oats, dates, cinnamon, and salt. Pulse until coarsely ground (be careful not to overprocess or you will end up with nut butter). Transfer to a medium mixing bowl and stir in the egg and vanilla.

3. Form the dough into golf ball–size balls, then flatten each ball slightly and place in the center of the mini pie or muffin pans. Use your fingers to press the dough evenly across the bottom and up the sides. Bake in the center of the oven for 10 minutes.

4. *To make the filling:* In a medium mixing bowl, combine the fruit, sugar, lemon juice, tapioca starch or cornstarch, cinnamon, and cardamom or nutmeg (if using).

5. Divide the filling among the crusts, piling the fruit high.

6. Bake in the center of the oven until the fruit softens and the crusts are lightly browned, 20 to 25 minutes.

7. Allow the pies to cool completely before removing. Run a knife around the edges to loosen and gently lift out.

TIP

Tapioca starch, also called tapioca flour, is a natural thickener that soaks up the juices in the fruit to prevent the crusts from getting soggy.

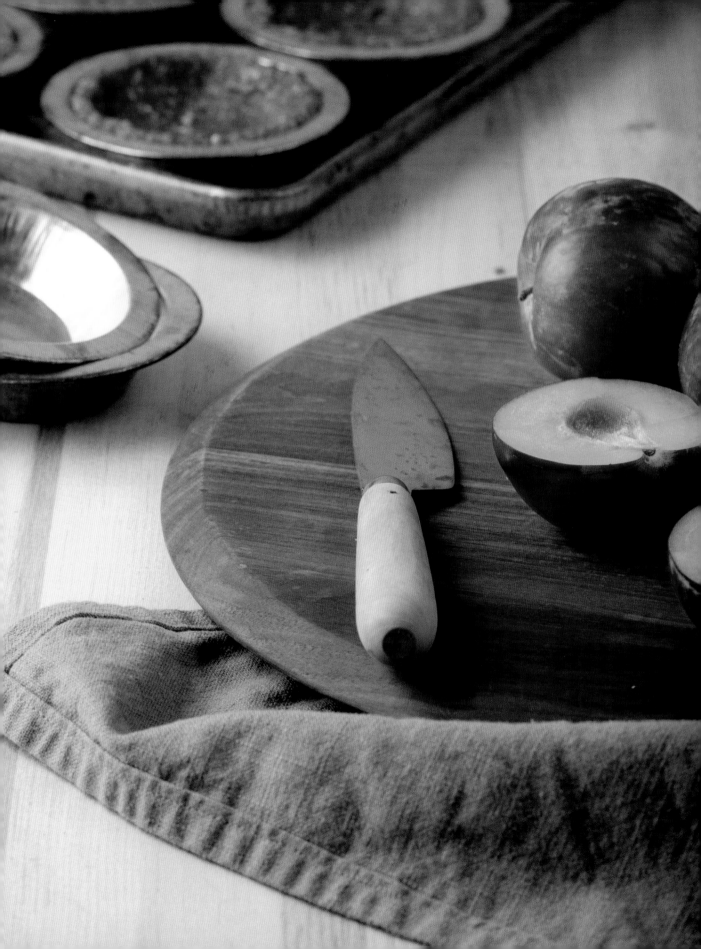

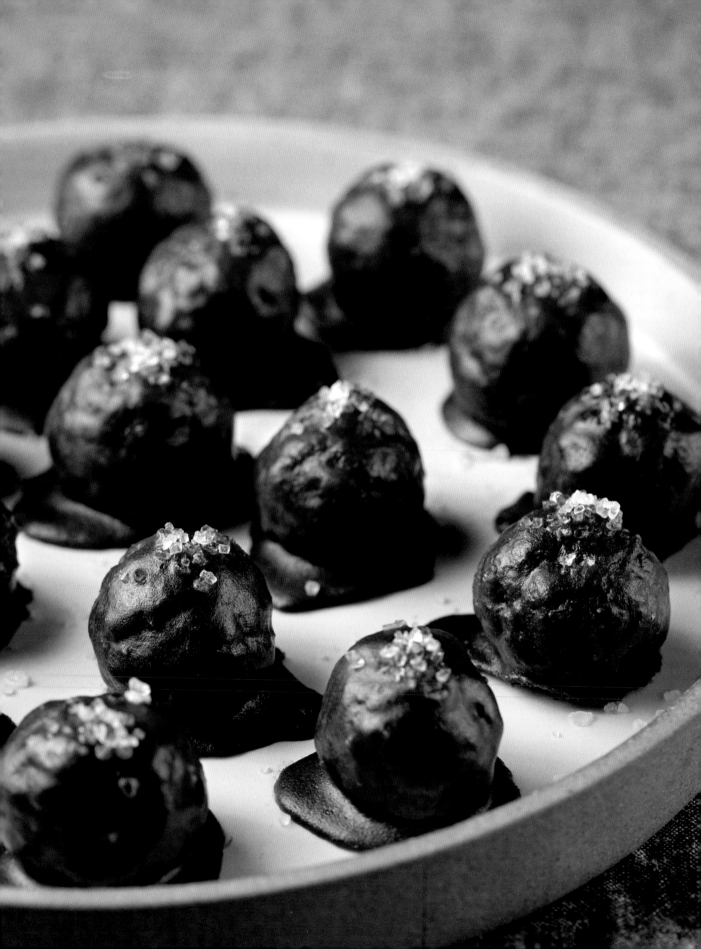

PECAN BUTTER CHOCOLATE TRUFFLES WITH SEA SALT

MAKES 18 BITE-SIZE TRUFFLES

for satisfying a sweet tooth

We happily classify dark chocolate as a health food (it's loaded with antioxidants), but store-bought chocolate treats are loaded with refined sugar and hydrogenated oils, both of which obliterate the health benefits. Fear not! Shalane's got your back. She requested that Elyse come up with a crave-worthy chocolate treat free of refined sugar, and these incredible vegan truffle babies were born.

First, you make the sweet, cinnamon-laced pecan butter. (Make a double batch—it's almost impossible not to eat by the spoonful right out of the bowl.) Then you roll it into balls. Finally, you dip each ball in the simple chocolate coating.

FOR THE PECAN BUTTER

2 cups pecans

10 Deglet dates, pitted

½ teaspoon ground cinnamon

FOR THE COATING

2 tablespoons virgin coconut oil

3 tablespoons maple syrup

3 tablespoons unsweetened cocoa powder

1 teaspoon coarse sea salt

1. Preheat the oven to 350°F. Line a baking sheet with parchment paper.

2. *To make the pecan butter:* Spread the pecans out on a baking sheet and roast in the center of the oven for 8 minutes, stirring after 4 minutes. Allow the pecans to cool completely.

3. In a food processor or high-speed blender, combine the pecans, dates, and cinnamon. Pulse or blend on high until smooth, stopping as needed to scrape underneath the blade. (Do not overprocess—you want the pecan butter to be thick.) Transfer to a small bowl.

4. Use your hands to roll the pecan butter into bite-size balls. (If the nut butter is warm or liquid-y, chill it in the fridge to make it easier to handle.) Place the balls on the baking sheet.

5. *To make the coating:* Place the oil in a small microwaveable bowl and microwave in increments of 10 seconds, stirring in between, until almost completely melted. (Alternatively, the oil can be melted in a small saucepan over low heat.) Stir in the maple syrup and cocoa powder until smooth.

6. Drop one ball at a time in the chocolate coating, use a fork to lift out, and return to the baking sheet. Continue with the remaining balls. Top each truffle with a small pinch of the salt.

7. Place the baking sheet in the fridge for 10 to 15 minutes or until ready to serve. Use a spatula to transfer to a serving plate.

8. Store leftovers in an airtight container, lined with parchment paper, in the fridge for up to 1 week or in the freezer for up to 3 months.

BAKED MOUNT HOOD APPLES

SERVES 4

for keeping the doc away

If you have leftover unfiltered apple juice, use it make our Apple-Ginger Cider (page 39), then warm up with a mug of it.

Come fall, one of our favorite pastimes is a day trip to the farms in Hood River, at the base of Mount Hood, to ramble through the orchards and pick endless varieties of apples. We always come home with more apples than we know what to do with. For a simple, homey dessert, we like to bake the apples whole and stuff them with nuts, cinnamon, and butter, of course.

Apples are a stellar food for athletes since they're blood-sugar regulators, inflammation fighters, and cardiovascular strengtheners. Eat the skin for the maximum benefits.

---

4 apples (Granny Smith, Honeycrisp, or Pink Lady)

½ cup chopped pecans or walnuts

¼ cup dark amber maple syrup

1 teaspoon ground cinnamon

¼ teaspoon ground cardamom or ground ginger (optional)

¼ teaspoon fine sea salt

1 tablespoon cold unsalted butter, cut into 4 pieces

1 cup unfiltered apple juice

Vanilla ice cream (optional)

1. Preheat the oven to 375°F.

2. Use an apple corer to remove the core of each apple and widen the opening slightly larger. Place the apples in an 8 x 8-inch baking dish.

3. In a small bowl, mix together the nuts, maple syrup, cinnamon, cardamom or ginger (if using), and salt. Spoon the filling into each apple, packing them to the brim. Top each apple with a piece of butter.

4. Pour the apple juice into the bottom of the baking dish.

5. Place in the center of the oven and bake until tender but not mushy, 35 to 45 minutes. Halfway through baking, spoon some of the juice over each apple.

6. Place each apple in individual bowls. Carefully pour the juice from the bottom of the dish into a small saucepan and simmer, uncovered, on low until it reduces by half, about 10 minutes. Split the apples open and pour the juice generously over top.

7. Serve warm with a scoop of vanilla ice cream (if desired).

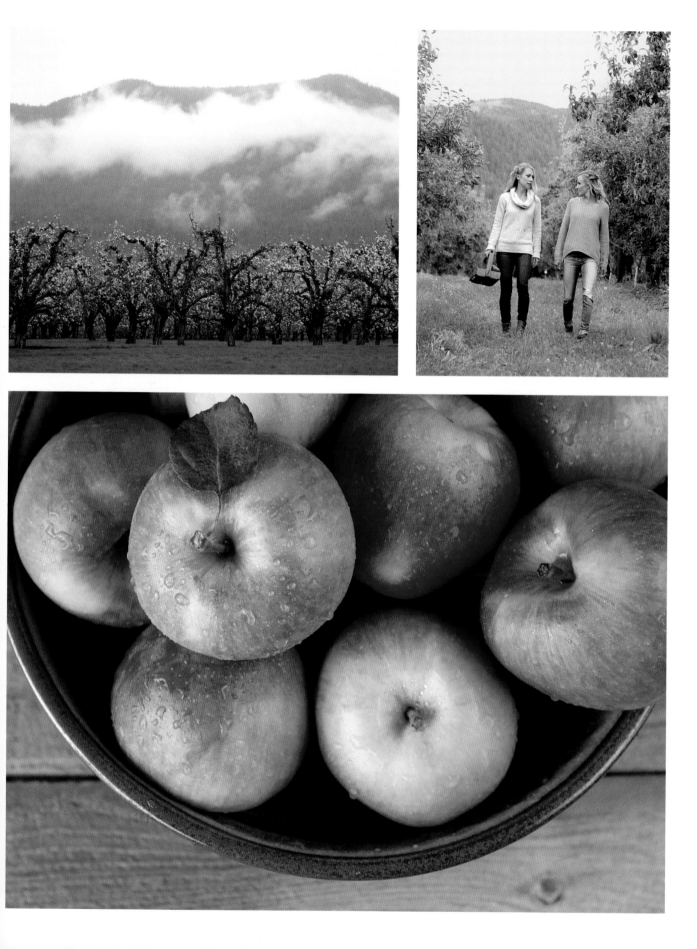

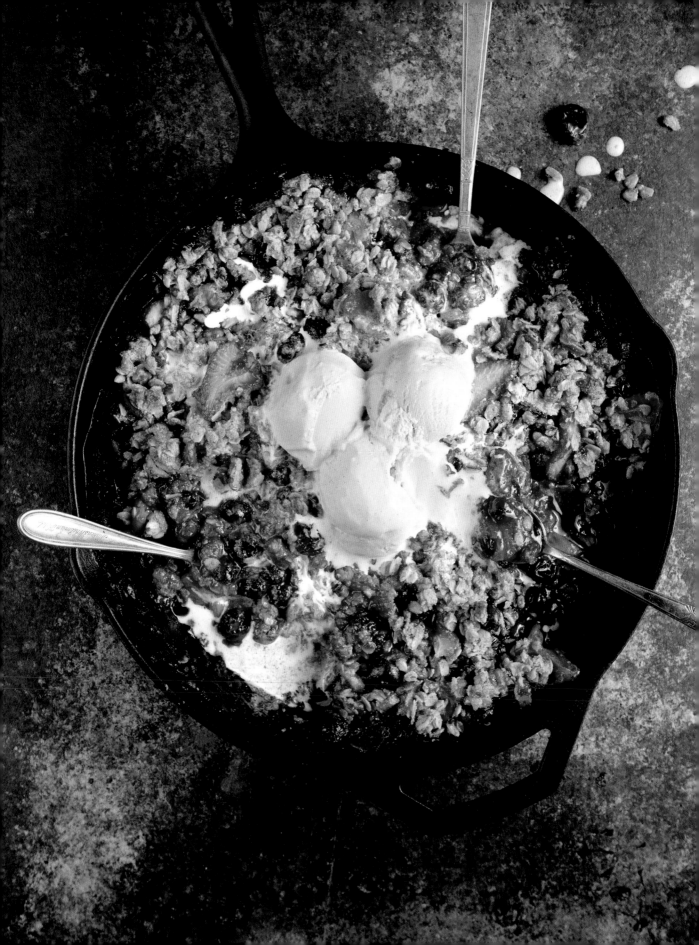

OREGON BERRY CRUMBLE

SERVES 5

for wholesome happiness

Since everyone will want seconds and the leftovers are delicious for breakfast with a scoop of yogurt, we highly recommend doubling the recipe and baking it in a 9 x 13-inch baking dish.

This is Elyse's favorite recipe from her childhood. We tweaked it to make it more wholesome and free of cane sugar, flour, and dairy. And we promise we aren't just saying this, but we like the taste of this gluten-free, vegan-friendly variation even better.

Come winter, this recipe can be made with frozen berries, but berries picked at their peak of sweetness are preferable. Every summer we pick local Oregon berries at Sauvie Island and stockpile our freezers.

The fruit is tossed with all-natural tapioca flour, also known as tapioca starch, to absorb excess moisture from the fruit, but cornstarch can also be used.

---

3 cups sliced strawberries

3 cups blueberries

1 tablespoon lemon juice

2 tablespoons tapioca flour or tapioca starch

¾ cup old-fashioned rolled oats (gluten-free if sensitive)

½ cup almond flour or almond meal

½ cup chopped raw walnuts or pecans

½ teaspoon ground cinnamon

¼ teaspoon ground ginger

¼ teaspoon fine sea salt

⅓ cup grade B maple syrup

¼ cup virgin coconut oil, melted

Vanilla ice cream (coconut milk-based if sensitive to dairy), optional

1. Preheat the oven to 400°F. Place an 8 x 8-inch baking dish, a 10-inch skillet, or 6 small ramekins (ovenproof individual-serving bowls) on a baking sheet.

2. In a large bowl, toss together the strawberries, blueberries, lemon juice, and tapioca flour or starch. Spread the mixture in the baking dish or skillet, or divide among the ramekins and pack them as full as possible.

3. In the same bowl, whisk together the oats, almond flour or meal, nuts, cinnamon, ginger, and salt. Add the maple syrup and oil and stir until combined.

4. Spread the oat topping evenly over the berry mixture.

5. Place in the center of the oven. Bake until the topping is golden brown and the fruit is bubbling, 25 to 30 minutes (20 minutes if using ramekins). If the berries were frozen, add an extra 10 minutes.

6. Serve warm or at room temperature with a scoop of vanilla ice cream (if desired).

COCOA-COCONUT MACAROONS

MAKES 2 DOZEN

for squelching a sweet tooth

 Dress them up by drizzling melted chocolate over top and sprinkling with crushed pistachios.

Okay, first a disclaimer: These cookie bites are gluten-free, refined sugar-free, egg-free, and flour-free. Wait, don't skip to the next page. They're also incredibly rich and lusciously sweet and will squelch even the most problematic sweet tooth. And since you can count the main ingredients on one hand, they're the easiest coconut macaroon recipe you'll ever find.

Since shredded coconut comes in many different sizes, weighing the coconut will give you the most accurate measurement. If you're using an already finely shredded brand of coconut like Bob's Red Mill, you do not need to pulse the coconut further and only need 2¼ cups. For this recipe, we used 3 cups of Trader Joe's unsweetened flaked coconut, which requires pulsing in a food processor to get the right consistency.

---

7 ounces (2¼ to 3 cups, depending on brand) unsweetened shredded dried coconut (see headnote above)

¼ cup unsweetened cocoa powder

¼ teaspoon fine sea salt

½ cup maple syrup

2 tablespoons virgin coconut oil, melted

2 teaspoons vanilla extract

1. Preheat the oven to 325°F. Line a baking sheet with parchment paper.

2. In a food processor or high-speed blender, pulse the coconut until it's the consistency of coarse sand. Transfer to a large mixing bowl and stir in the cocoa powder and salt. Add the maple syrup, oil, and vanilla and stir until combined.

3. Press the dough into a tablespoon measuring spoon and drop onto the baking sheet. Bake until crisp on the outside and soft in the middle, 20 minutes.

4. Allow the macaroons to cool completely before transferring to a plate or storing in an airtight container.

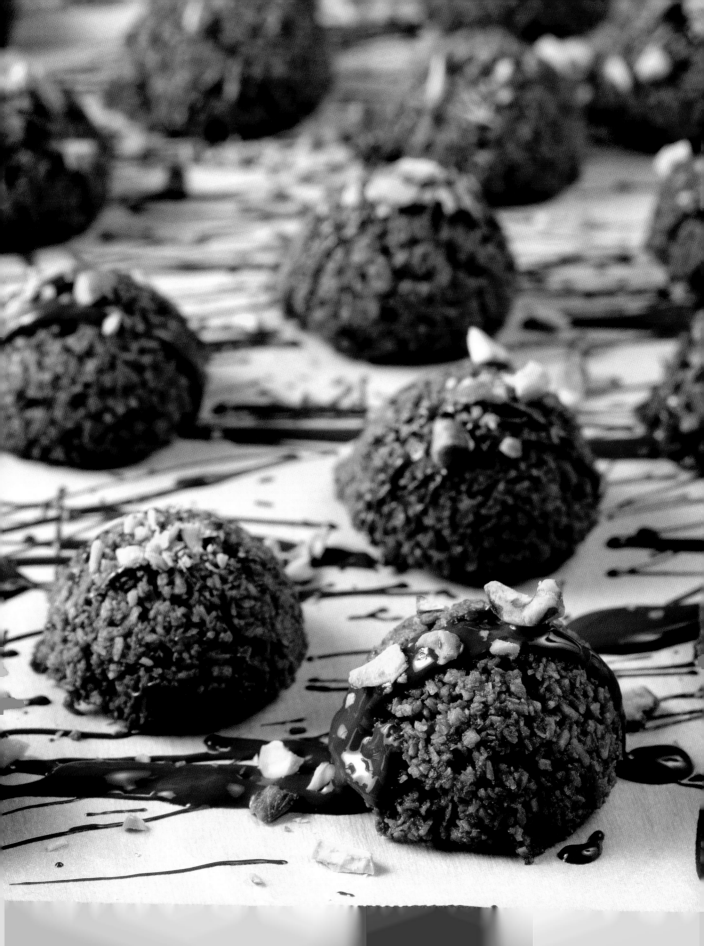

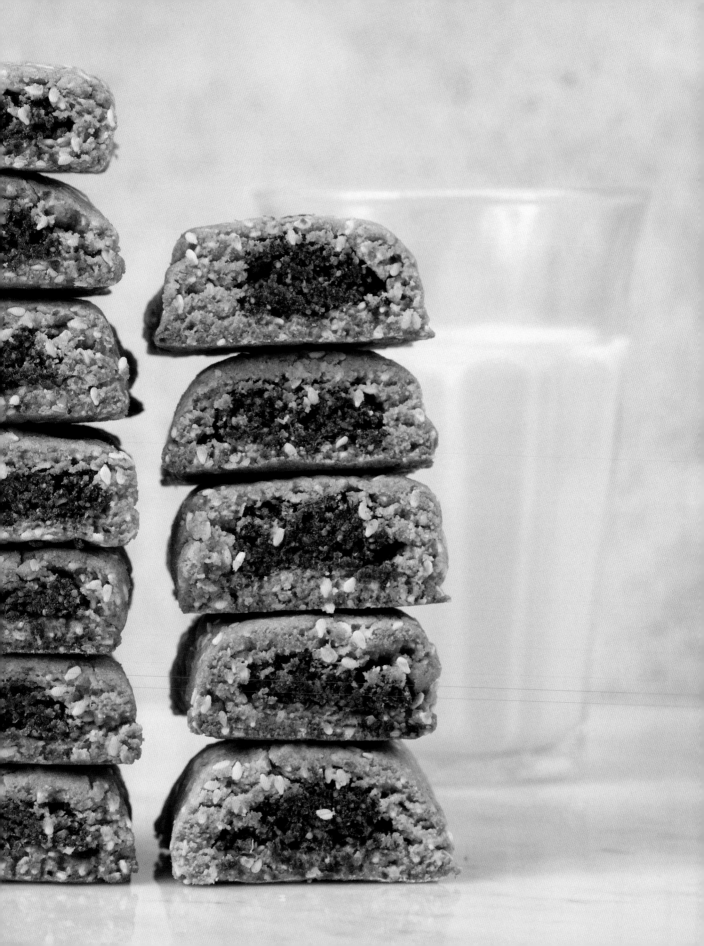

FIG JAM COOKIES

MAKES 24 COOKIES

for wholesome energy

FILLING

2 cups (10 ounces) dried black mission figs, stems removed

⅓ cup tahini (ground sesame seeds)

1 tablespoon water

2 teaspoons ground cinnamon

DOUGH

1½ cups whole wheat flour

1 cup almond flour or almond meal

½ cup sesame seeds

½ teaspoon fine sea salt

⅓ cup coconut oil

½ cup maple syrup

1 teaspoon vanilla extract

These fig-and-tahini-stuffed cookies are 10 times better than the Fig Newtons of our childhood. We recall bringing packages of those soft, fig-filled cookies to track meets because we thought they were healthy. But a look at the list of ingredients is alarming— high-fructose corn syrup, partially hydrogenated cottonseed oil, artificial flavor, preservatives, and a few other ingredients that we aren't sure how to pronounce. Yikes.

Our own fat little fig cookies, despite being sweet, won't cause a blood sugar spike and crash since they're perfectly balanced with fiber from the figs and healthy fats from the sesame seeds, almond flour, and coconut oil. They're also road-tested. Shalane gave these cookies rave reviews as an energizing snack before her p.m. runs (yes, Shalane's training regimen often includes two runs a day— once in the morning, then again in the afternoon!).

These cookies take time to prepare since you have to make the filling and roll out the dough, but they're a fun, rainy day activity.

1. Preheat the oven to 350°F. Line a baking sheet with parchment paper.

2. *To make the filling:* In a food processor, combine the figs, tahini, water, and cinnamon and puree until smooth, stopping as needed to scrape down the sides and underneath the blade.

3. *To make the dough:* In a large bowl, whisk together the whole wheat flour, almond flour or meal, sesame seeds, and salt.

4. Place the oil in a small microwaveable bowl and microwave in increments of 10 seconds, stirring in between, until almost completely melted. (Alternatively, the oil can be melted in a small saucepan over low heat.) Stir in the maple syrup and vanilla. Pour over the flour mixture and mix until a dough forms.

(continued)

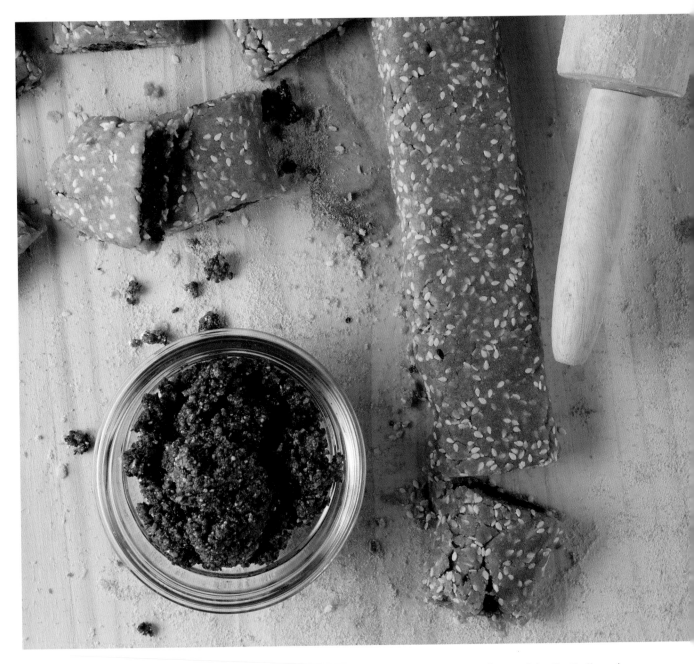

5. *To form the cookies:* Divide the dough into 3 balls. Roll each ball out on a lightly floured work surface to create three 12 x 4-inch rectangles (use your hands to shape while rolling). Divide the fig jam into thirds, shape into 1-inch wide logs, and place centered on each piece of dough. Fold the edges of the dough over the figs to overlap slightly in the middle and press gently to seal (use your fingers to smooth out any cracks).

6. Gently roll the tops of each log to slightly flatten. Slice each log into 8 cookies and bake until lightly golden, 15 to 20 minutes. Transfer to a rack to cool.

MANGO-RASPBERRY-BASIL FROZEN YOGURT

SERVES 4

for a refreshing frozen treat

To make this recipe dairy-free and vegan, substitute 1 cup canned unsweetened coconut milk for the yogurt.

The three fruits Shalane craves are mangoes, raspberries, and bananas. We decided to take two of her favorites and combine them with whole milk yogurt and a touch of fresh basil to create this tongue-tingling frozen treat.

Unlike store-bought sorbet or frozen yogurt, we let the fruit shine and don't overpower it with cane sugar. Our frozen yogurt is lightly sweetened with a touch of maple syrup.

No fancy ice cream maker is required to whirl this dessert together. All you'll need is a blender and 5 minutes tops.

1 cup frozen mango chunks

1 cup frozen raspberries

1 cup plain whole milk yogurt

¼ cup maple syrup

10 basil leaves

3 tablespoons chia seeds (optional)

1. In a high-speed blender, place the mango, raspberries, yogurt, maple syrup, basil, and chia seeds (if using). Blend until smooth.

2. Serve immediately or transfer to a freezer-safe container and freeze for up to 3 months. If frozen, take out of the freezer 20 to 30 minutes prior to serving, to soften.

DARK CHOCOLATE-DIPPED BANANA POPS

MAKES 6 POPS

for satisfying an ice cream craving

We've been dipping frozen bananas in melted chocolate since our college days (yes, we runners have odd habits!). If you've never eaten a frozen banana, you gotta try it. Its consistency transforms into that of ice cream.

We have since happily discovered that they're even better dipped in our homemade chocolate sauce, a magical combination of unsweetened cocoa powder, coconut oil, and maple syrup. Since our banana pops are now free of refined sugar, we think this qualifies them for the podium.

If you're sensitive to dairy but are struggling to give up beloved ice cream, this recipe is for you!

3 ripe bananas, peeled and cut in half widthwise

¼ cup virgin coconut oil

⅓ cup maple syrup

6 tablespoons unsweetened cocoa powder

½ cup finely chopped roasted nuts or shredded coconut

1. Cut 3 wooden skewers in half and insert a skewer lengthwise through the middle of each banana. Place the 6 banana pops on a plate and freeze for at least 4 hours or overnight.

2. Place the oil in a low-sided microwaveable bowl and microwave on low in increments of 10 seconds, stirring in between, until almost completely melted. (Alternatively, the oil can be melted in a small saucepan over low heat.) Stir in the maple syrup and cocoa powder.

3. Roll one banana at a time in the chocolate coating to completely cover and immediately sprinkle with the nuts or coconut. Set the chocolate-covered bananas back on the plate. If the chocolate in the bowl begins to solidify, you may need to warm it again.

4. Keep the bananas in the freezer until ready to serve, or transfer to a gallon-size freezer bag and store for up to 3 months.

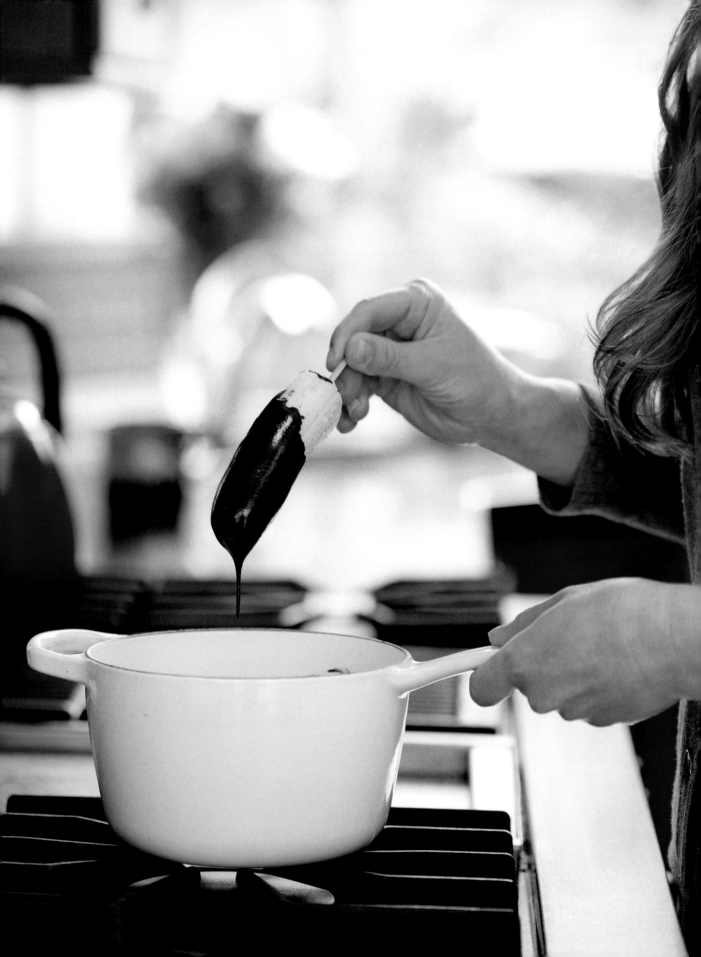

SWEET CINNAMON TAHINI BUTTER

MAKES ¾ CUP

for a calcium-rich spread

Make your own tahini paste to use in hummus (page 70), salad dressing (page 173), and soup (page 102). Hulled sesame seeds work best for these uses. Simply grind a cup or two of toasted hulled sesame seeds in a food processor until smooth.

If you eat as much nut butter as we do, you might be ready to mix it up—or if you have a nut allergy, this recipe is for you! This cinnamon-speckled, honey-sweetened butter is made from whole (unhulled) sesame seeds. Freshly grinding your own seeds results in a more nutritious butter since there's a hearty dose of good stuff like calcium in the hull (store-bought tahini is made from hulled seeds).

Unhulled sesame seeds can be found in the bulk bins at most grocery stores. The texture of this butter is thick and is best for spreading on hearty whole grain toast. Make a double batch. It won't last long.

---

1 cup raw unhulled sesame seeds

2 tablespoons virgin coconut oil

¼ teaspoon fine sea salt

2 tablespoons honey

2 teaspoons ground cinnamon

1. Heat a dry cast-iron skillet over medium heat. Add the seeds and toast until fragrant, stirring frequently, about 5 minutes (being careful not to let them brown). Set the seeds aside to cool.

2. In a food processor, process the sesame seeds on high until they form a chunky paste, 2 to 3 minutes. Add the oil and salt and process until smooth, 1 to 2 minutes. Add the honey and cinnamon and pulse briefly until combined.

3. Transfer to a glass jar and store in the fridge for up to 1 month. To make it easier to spread, take out from the fridge 15 minutes prior to using.

4. Serve smeared on thick slices of whole grain toast.

COFFEE-VANILLA PEANUT BUTTER

MAKES 3 CUPS

for focus and stamina

For the nuttiest flavor, buy your peanuts raw and roast them yourself at 350°F for 25 to 30 minutes, stirring after 15 minutes. Make sure they are completely cool prior to blending.

Add a tablespoon or two of maca powder, ground flax, or chia seeds to give this butter superpowers.

This recipe comes to us from our friend Jen Huntington, a fellow UNC Tar Heel, who after college went on to study nutrition and started her own nut butter company called Huntington Provision Co. When we heard she was making peanut butter with coffee, we were intrigued and begged her to reveal the recipe. One spoonful of this peanut butter stuck on the roofs of our mouths, and we knew we had to put her recipe in our book.

Jen told us that in college she was inspired by Shalane's focus, strength, and toughness when it came to facing a challenge. Funny enough, we think this peanut butter has matching attributes. Try a smear of it on a banana before your a.m. run and you'll feel the focused stamina.

4 cups unsalted roasted peanuts

⅔ cup coconut sugar or other granulated sugar

2 tablespoons freshly ground coffee

1 tablespoon coconut oil, slightly melted, or olive oil

1 tablespoon vanilla extract

1 teaspoon fine sea salt (leave out if peanuts are salted)

1. Place the peanuts in a food processor or high-speed blender. Process or blend until there are no visible pieces of nuts and it begins to look smooth (be careful not to overprocess or you'll end up with a peanut liquid instead of butter).

2. Add the sugar, coffee, oil, vanilla, and salt and blend just until incorporated.

3. For a longer shelf life and to prevent oil separation, store in a glass jar in the fridge for up to 6 months. Leave out at room temperature for 15 minutes prior to devouring, to make it easier to spread.

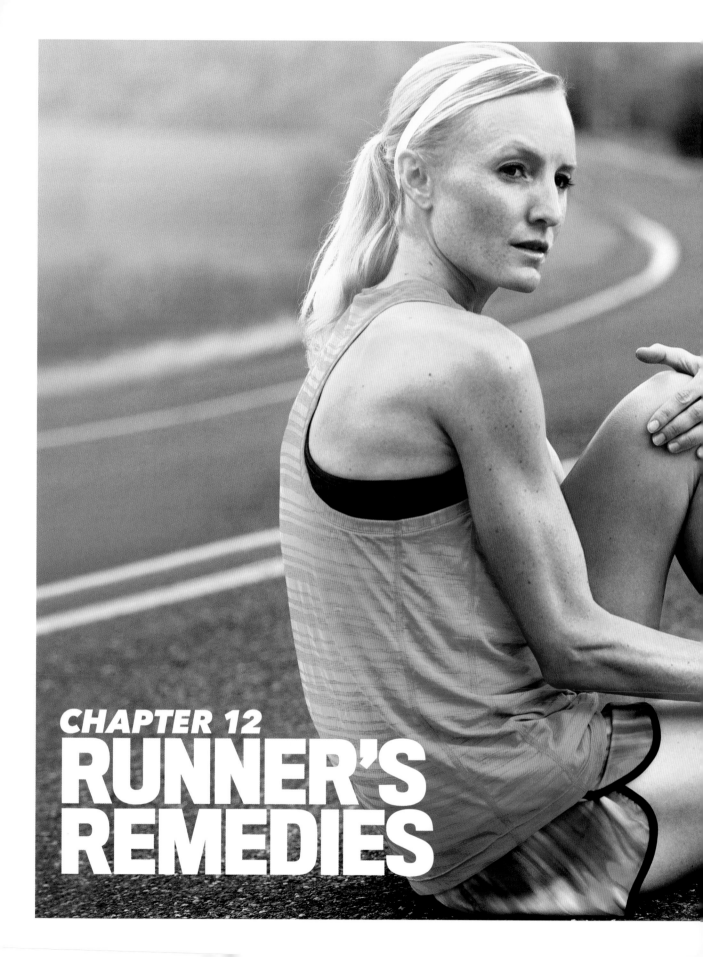

CHAPTER 12
RUNNER'S REMEDIES

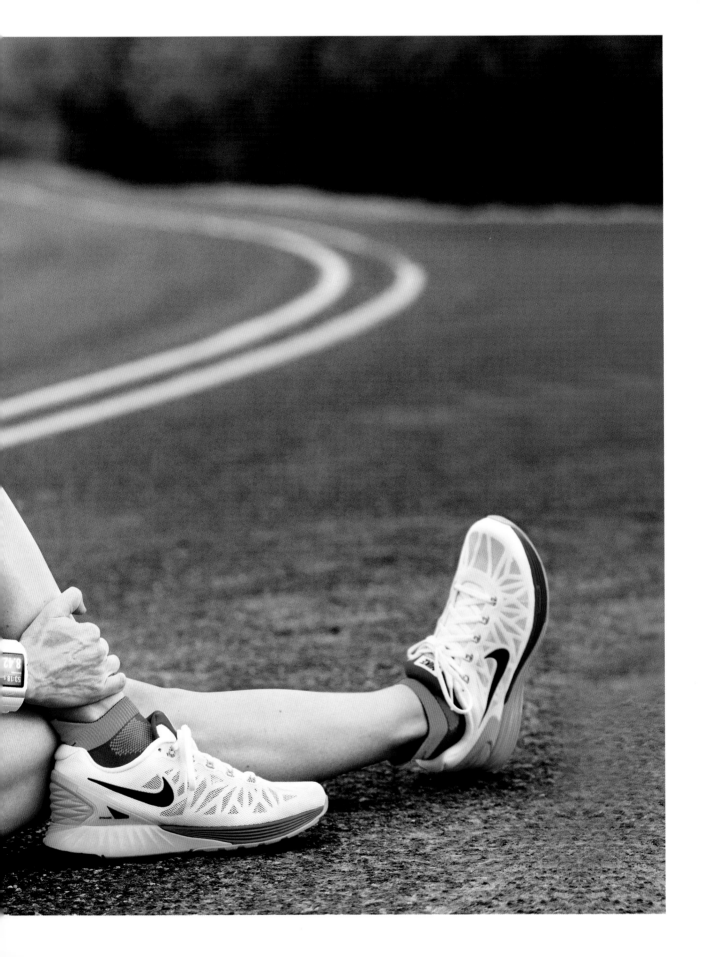

Most runners don't look to the kitchen when struggling with an injury or illness. But the kitchen is the first place you should turn to when dealing with common running ailments. Nourishing food can be a runner's first line of defense for preventing and overcoming common aches and pains. (However, when dealing with medical concerns or injuries, please consult with a doctor.)

In this chapter, we reveal our home-brewed solutions for fighting anemia, athletic amenorrhea, burnout and stress, colds and flu, dehydration, digestive distress, inflammation, muscle aches, and stress fractures.

In the words of Shalane, "I'd rather eat my way to health."

ANEMIA

Anemia is a deficiency of red blood cells in the body and is most often caused by low iron levels. Red blood cells are critical to athletes since their role is to transport oxygen to your hardworking muscles. An adequate supply of iron must be available to assist this process. Mild anemia can impact athletic performance since it causes a general feeling of tiredness.

Anemia is most common in women with heavy menstrual cycles, vegetarians, and athletes training at a high level. If you're concerned you might be anemic, you should have your levels checked. To restore iron levels, you may need to take a supplement, but since it's possible to overdose on iron, it's best to consult with a doctor.

Also, iron isn't the only nutrient needed to overcome anemia. It works optimally in conjunction with other nutrients including vitamins B_{12}, C, and A, which occur together naturally in many whole foods.

Our top devour-worthy foods for overcoming low iron stores include red meat, dark meat chicken, dark leafy greens, dried fruit (raisins, dates, apricots, figs), nuts, sesame seeds, seaweed, beans, cumin, oregano, molasses, beets, and tomatoes.

RECIPES FOR PREVENTING ANEMIA

ATHLETIC AMENORRHEA

Athletic amenorrhea is the absence of menstruation in female athletes due to low estrogen levels, which is caused by the combination of high-energy expenditure and inadequate nutritional intake. It is most common in distance runners and ballet dancers. It can be caused by disordered eating habits, but in many cases it's simply a lack of the right fuel. If not treated, it can lead to serious long-term health concerns including infertility and osteoporosis.

Elyse experienced athletic amenorrhea firsthand throughout high school and college and suffered from stress fractures due to low bone density. Doctors told her that she'd have trouble getting pregnant someday, but not a single doctor suggested she change her diet. Luckily, Elyse discovered a passion for cooking, and when she began introducing more fat into her diet, her estrogen levels returned to normal. Long story short—she now has a beautiful baby girl.

Getting more high-quality calories into the diet is the best line of defense. A diet rich in healthy fats is essential for maintaining hormone health in female athletes. And a high intake of minerals and vitamins from whole food sources—including folic acid, zinc, iron, magnesium, calcium, and vitamins A, B, C, and E—is critical.

The best calorie-dense whole foods to fuel up on include nuts, seeds, salmon, sardines, dark meat chicken, beef (yes, even the saturated fat in grass-fed meat is healthy), whole milk yogurt, butter, eggs, olive oil, coconut oil, and avocados.

All the recipes in this book are nutrient-dense and can greatly help someone suffering from athletic amenorrhea and/or eating disorders. We hope our passion for "indulgent nourishment" shows young female athletes everywhere that food is not only fuel but also meant to be enjoyed.

RECIPES FOR OVERCOMING AMENORRHEA

BURNOUT, LOW ENERGY, STRESS, IRRITABILITY

If you're in the midst of intense training and find yourself feeling drained, stressed, and irritable, you may be running on empty, which can lead to feeling "hangry" all the time. When you're pushing your body to its limit, you need an incredible amount of nourishment to keep your systems working optimally. This nourishment can be tough to get if you're relying on nutrient-poor processed foods, sugar, and/or caffeine to get through your day.

Hormones, which control everything from our mood to our metabolism, need fuel to function optimally. If you're feeling depleted, you may simply just not be getting enough high-quality calories in your diet from healthy fats and complex carbohydrates. You also need plenty of B vitamins, which are essential for converting food into energy. Feeling tired could also be a sign that your iron stores are low (see "Anemia" on page 208).

The best energy-giving whole foods to prevent burning out include meat, legumes, whole grains, and vegetables for their balanced macronutrients and range of B vitamins. If you're eating a varied diet, you're likely getting enough B vitamins since they're in a broad range of whole foods. Vegans and vegetarians might have trouble getting enough vitamin B and should include tempeh and sea vegetables in their diet.

If you're feeling stressed to the max, your adrenal system might be tapped out. You need the right nourishment to support your adrenal system, and here again B vitamins are essential. Vitamin D, the sunshine vitamin, is also critical. Many Americans are low on D since we spend so much time indoors. Getting sunshine and fresh air first thing in the a.m. can significantly boost your mood.

Green tea is a fabulous drink for a boost of antioxidants and energy. Unlike coffee, green tea provides even energy instead of a high followed by a crash. Dates are a fabulous whole food source of glucose for a quick boost before a hard workout. And here's the best part. Chocolate, thanks to its rich flavonoids, helps fight fatigue and depression and provides support to the adrenal system. Dark chocolate with at least 70 percent cocoa content might be your new BFF.

RECIPES FOR ENERGY AND COMBATING STRESS

COLDS AND FLU

When cold and flu season rolls around, your best line of defense is immune-boosting whole foods, adequate rest, sunshine for vitamin D, staying hydrated, and managing stress. To up your immune-fighting cells, fill your basket with a broad range of fruits and veggies.

The best foods to boost the immune system include vitamin C-rich citrus; antioxidant-loaded berries; phytonutrient-loving vegetables; zinc-rich nuts and seeds; probiotic foods like fermented veggies, miso, and yogurt; and foods with antibacterial and antiviral properties, including raw garlic and coconut.

Our favorite flu-fighting dishes are soups and stews since they're hydrating, comforting, and nourishing, all in one bowl. The soups in this cookbook pack a mean punch of veggies and never skimp on garlic. Garlic is such a fabulous immune booster that at the first sign of illness, Elyse takes a "garlic-honey shot," which is simply a spoonful of minced raw garlic coated in honey to make it easier to swallow. Shalane once tried this remedy right before heading out on a run and wasn't a fan of the garlic burps, but it did the trick. She didn't get sick.

RECIPES TO BOOST THE IMMUNE SYSTEM

DEHYDRATION

Restoring fluids lost during an intense sweat session sometimes calls for more than just sipping water. That's because plain water lacks the electrolytes necessary to restore your body's fluid balance. While sports drinks are a great source of electrolytes, they're also full of ingredients we don't love, including artificial flavors and colors, high-fructose corn syrup, and/or artificial sweeteners.

Luckily you can get plenty of electrolytes from more natural drinks and whole foods. Our favorite drinks for hydrating before and during an intense workout include coconut water, 100% pure cranberry juice, or fresh-squeezed orange juice, all diluted with filtered water. If you need an extra glucose boost during a workout, blending the drink with a few dates or a tablespoon of maple syrup and a pinch of high-quality sea salt will do the trick. After a workout, our drinks of choice include coconut water diluted with sparkling mineral water and a squeeze of fresh lemon juice or any of our favorite homemade beverages and smoothies listed below.

Post-sweat it's essential to restore sodium, potassium, calcium, and magnesi33um levels, which all help the body retain fluids. Whole foods rich in these crucial minerals include bananas, oranges, coconuts, walnuts, vegetables (sea vegetables are especially mineral-rich), sweet potatoes, miso paste, Parmesan, and high-quality sea salt (learn more about the minerals in sea salt on page 15). Even on a hot day, soup is incredibly hydrating since it provides needed fluids, salt, and minerals all in one package.

RECIPES TO PREVENT DEHYDRATION

DIGESTIVE DISTRESS

One look at the line in front of the porta-potties at a road race and it's apparent that digestive distress is a common problem among runners. That's because when you run, your body prioritizes oxygen flow to your muscles at the expense of oxygenating other systems like digestion.

A healthy digestive system is critical to ensure you're able to absorb the maximum amount of nutrients from the healthy food you're devouring. Everyone reacts differently to foods, so the best way to learn what could be causing discomfort is to keep a food journal. Common culprits of an upset tummy include dairy, gluten, and sugar. Also what you're not eating could be just as much of the problem as what you are eating.

The best foods to include in your diet to boost digestion are raw salads, which are rich in digestion-enhancing enzymes; probiotic-rich foods like miso, kimchi, kombucha, sauerkraut, apple cider vinegar, and yogurt; alkalizing foods like lemon juice in warm water; and just the right amount of fiber (enough to keep things moving but not too fast!).

Slowing down and taking the time to chew your food instead of eating while on the go especially helps get the digestive juices flowing. Staying hydrated throughout the day is also essential. Lastly, there are amazing foods that help soothe the intestinal tract. Best bets include homemade bone broth, chia seeds, ginger, tropical fruit like pineapple and mango, and soothing herbs like fennel seeds, mint, and cardamom.

Our favorite easy-to-digest complex carbohydrates for carbo-loading the night before a big race are sweet potatoes and rice. The fastest digesting fats are medium-chain fatty acids like coconut oil. And our favorite easy-to-digest proteins are chicken and fish. You should never try anything new right before a race. Find what foods work best for you by experimenting throughout your training.

RECIPES TO IMPROVE DIGESTION

INFLAMMATION

Many of the most common running injuries—including Achilles tendinitis, runner's knee, plantar fasciitis, shin splints, hip pain, and iliotibial band syndrome—are caused by chronic inflammation from overuse without proper recovery. Instead of popping pills for pain, reach for foods with natural anti-inflammatory compounds and healing properties.

Our top picks for fighting inflammation include herbs, spices, olive oil, fish, nuts, seeds, oats, avocado, beets, and berries. Studies show 2 tablespoons of olive oil has as much of an anti-inflammatory effect as one dose of ibuprofen, and it's definitely more fun to eat. Spices, thanks to their anti-inflammatory properties, are incredible healing foods. Our podium winners are ginger, cinnamon, and turmeric (you'll find these spices frequently in our recipes).

Lastly, when it comes to inflammation, what you're not eating is just as important as what you are eating. The Standard American Diet is high in sugar, dairy, and omega-6 fatty acids (from vegetable oils), all of which cause inflammation. To balance out the omega-6 in our diets, foods rich in omega-3 fatty acids are essential.

RECIPES TO FIGHT INFLAMMATION

MUSCLE ACHES AND RECOVERY

Food repairs muscles after an intense training session. The right foods can greatly help speed up recovery time and reduce the aches and pains. Postworkout your body needs nutrient-dense foods to replace the minerals lost during sweat and protein-rich whole foods to rebuild muscles.

The best proteins for recovery are those that contain all nine essential amino acids. Sources include eggs (which have the highest net protein utilization, meaning they're easily assimilated), fish, and poultry. Plant-based protein-rich foods include nuts and seeds, beans, whole grains, tempeh, and quinoa. Magnesium can be especially beneficial for achy muscles, and calcium is essential for rebuilding bone mass.

Foods that are high in both magnesium and calcium include whole milk yogurt, dark leafy greens, whole grains, beans, fish, nuts and seeds, and dried fruit. A handful of nuts and dried fruit is an ideal snack to reach for postworkout to keep your body happy until dinner.

RECIPES FOR RECOVERY

STRESS FRACTURES

The human skeleton is made up of 206 bones. These bones are living organs in a constant state of change. Similarly to our muscles, exercise breaks down our bones, and nourished rest enables them to build back up. Therefore, our bones constantly need proper nutrition to maintain their strength.

Simply taking a calcium supplement is not the answer to strong bones. In fact, too much calcium can make the bones too hard and more brittle. When recovering from a stress fracture, filling up on nutrient-dense whole foods is your best bet to speed recovery. The essential nutrients for bone health include calcium, magnesium, vitamin D, and vitamin K. Also, adequate protein from a variety of sources and high-quality fats, especially omega-3 fatty acids, are paramount.

It's important to avoid the acid-forming foods that are so common in the Standard American Diet, including sugar, white flour, potatoes, white rice, trans fats, artificial sweeteners, and too much animal protein. These foods pull minerals out of the bones and can weaken them over time.

Our favorite foods for bone health include seaweed—which has 10 times the calcium of cow's milk—nuts and seeds, cauliflower, asparagus, leafy greens like kale and spinach (spinach should be cooked since it's high in oxalic acid), sardines, tempeh, beans, whole grains, eggs, whole milk yogurt, Parmesan, and (best of all) mineral-rich broths.

RECIPES FOR BONE HEALTH

Coconut-Kale Smoothie, page 31

Homemade Hazelnut Milk, page 34

Superhero Muffins, page 42

Swiss Muesli Bowl, page 46

On-the-Run Frittata Muffins, page 52

Arugula Cashew Pesto, page 67

Kale-Radicchio Salad with Farro, page 80

Omega Sardine Salad, page 94

Moroccan Lentil Salad with Cauliflower Couscous, page 96

Long Run Mineral Broth, page 111

Classic Chicken Bone Broth, page 113

Carrot-Ginger Soup, page 116

Miso Soup with Wakame, page 117

Garlicky Greens, page 164

Sweet Cinnamon Tahini Butter, page 204

APPENDIX A
CULINARY TIPS AND TOOLS

10 TIPS FOR HUNGRY RUNNERS

Cooking is a crucial life skill, a lost art form, and a gift that keeps on giving. Arguably it's as important as learning to read and write, but most schools no longer offer cooking classes and unfortunately very few of us cooked alongside our moms. For those who grew up with Sir Stouffer, Mr. Campbell, and Chef Boyardee in their kitchens, it's never too late to learn to cook.

Here are 10 tips to transform the beginner cook into a confident apron wearer.

1. Buy the freshest and highest quality ingredients you can get. Yes, it will cost you more, but the outcome will be far superior in both flavor and nutrition. Local, seasonal food requires little effort in the kitchen to transform into a dish that will bring everyone to the table.

    Buy spices in small quantities—or better yet, buy them whole and grind them fresh (an old coffee grinder works fabulous). Buy Parmesan in a big wedge and freshly grate just what you need. Squeeze lemon juice fresh. Chop your own vegetables and please don't buy those little jars of already minced garlic.

2. Don't fear salt. Salt is essential for drawing out the juices and flavors that transform ingredients and should be used every step of the way. You'll see in our recipes that we always add salt at the beginning of cooking, and we even include a small amount of salt in sweet treats. High-quality sea salt is an essential mineral (see page 15 to learn more) that athletes need. And your home-cooked food will still have far less sodium than packaged or restaurant foods. Keep a stash of fine sea salt in an easily accessible bowl next to the stove.

3. Don't fear fat. Fat is an essential component of cooking and is a carrier for flavor. A little fat can transform a dish from bland, dry, and boring to buttery, rich, and soul satisfying. And as you learned in Chapter 1, good fat is good for you.

4. Read through a recipe in its entirety before you begin and prep all the ingredients in advance. *Mise en place* is a French culinary phrase used by chefs the world over, and it literally means "putting in place." Put all your ingredients in place and the recipe will flow smoothly. You never want to leave oil unattended in a hot pan while you're scrambling to finish dicing the onion and carrots. The way an ingredient should be prepped appears beside its name in the ingredient list. Ingredients appear in order of usage.

5. Taste as you go (obviously don't taste meat dishes until they're fully cooked) and always taste your final masterpiece before serving it. If a dish tastes bland, it might need a little salt, a little more fat, a little acid to brighten the flavor (a splash of lemon juice or vinegar), more heat (add a pinch of red pepper flakes), or a touch of sweetener (if it's too acidic). Since

ingredients and cooking techniques vary tremendously, it's impossible to give precise measurements for seasonings. That's why we always leave it up to you to taste and decide if the dish needs any extra love.

6. Follow the recipe exactly as written the first time you make it, but then get creative with substitutions. Learn to cook with what you have on hand or what inspires you at the farmers' market. We offer seasonal substitutions when an ingredient can't be found year-round. Please never buy tomatoes in the winter—that is, unless you like the taste of cardboard.

7. Embrace leftovers as your best friend. If you're a time-starved parent, student on a budget, or always-hungry athlete, get in the habit of making double batches of recipes and freeze what you won't eat in a few days. Freeze in individual portions to make thawing easier.

   Soups, stews, sauces, beans, and grains freeze beautifully in zipper storage bags or containers with lids. If your family complains about eating the same dish two nights in a row, find creative ways to reinvent the dish. Leftover meat and veggies are delicious on top of a salad or sandwich.

8. Nominate Sunday or another non-workday as your culinary day to prep food for the week. Make a hearty grain salad with seasonal veggies for work lunches, roast a big tray of root veggies (leftover roasted veggies are fabulous in scrambled eggs or salads), prep fruits and vegetables for smoothies, bake a wholesome treat for healthy snacking, cook a pot of beans, roast a whole chicken, and make a batch of dressings or sauces to transform quick weeknight meals. (Mix and match on the above—we definitely don't expect you to accomplish all that in one day!)

9. Invest in high-quality kitchen tools and organize your kitchen so you can easily access this equipment. See the opposite page for a list of must-haves and nice-to-haves. A good knife is essential. Take a knife skills class or watch a few YouTube videos. You'll be thrilled to discover just how easy it can be to dice an onion or mince a clove of garlic. Stock your pantry while you're at it. See page 12 for an entire chapter dedicated to this.

10. Cooking is not a chore. Think of it as your new awesome hobby that benefits everyone in your life. Turn on music while you cook, open a bottle of wine, and enlist a family member or friend to help with the prep and cleanup. Have fun making mistakes—they'll likely still be edible (unless your disaster caused the fire alarm to go off!).

KITCHEN TOOLS

You don't need a lot to get started. Here are the essentials:

Large wooden cutting board and a second smaller board for fruit (so your fruit doesn't take on the essence of garlic—you'll be mincing a lot of garlic in this book)

Large saucepan

Large stockpot (6-quart or larger, for making broth and cooking pasta for a crowd)

Large skillet

Cooking utensils, including wooden spoon, rubber spatula, soup ladle, and metal spatula

Colander

Sieve with fine mesh (for rinsing grains and beans and for straining stock)

2 baking sheets (sheet pan)

Set of mixing bowls

Salad spinner

Can opener

Cheese grater

Vegetable peeler

Magnetic kitchen timer (stick it on your fridge and use religiously)

Glass jars in a variety of sizes

Pepper mill (always grind black pepper fresh)

Lemon/lime squeezer

Measuring cups and measuring spoons

And here are a few more kitchen favorites that are worth the investment. Put them on your holiday wish list.

8-inch chef's knife (the only knife you really need—okay, maybe a serrated bread knife, too, so you can buy crusty loaves)

Professional high-speed blender (top-quality blenders can be used for making everything from smoothies to energy bars to nut butters and soups)

Cast-iron skillet (gets better with age—learn how to care for it correctly to keep it well-seasoned)

French oven (large cast-iron pot with enamel coating and lid, like Le Creuset)

Stir-fry pan (large wok)

Ceramic baking dish (13 x 9-inch size, holds in more heat than glass and can go from oven to table)

Springform cake pan (removable sides, 9-inch)

Ceramic quiche/pie pan (9-inch)

Slow cooker

Immersion blender (stick blender)

RESOURCES

WHERE TO SHOP

All the unusual ingredients in this book can be found at your local natural foods store or online at the following sites.

Bobsredmill.com: Whole grains, flours, legumes

Edenfoods.com: Top-quality organic ingredients

Fettlebotanic.com: Herbal teas, dried herbs

Great-eastern-sun.com: Asian-style condiments, dried seaweed (such as dulse, kombu), and miso

Pmrbuffalo.com: Our favorite local grass-fed meats

Spectrumorganics.com: Top-quality cooking oils

Thrivemarket.com: Organic products at wholesale prices

Online Resources

Eat Well Guide: Find local, sustainable food
eatwellguide.org

Eat Wild: Find sources for local food and grass-fed meat and dairy
eatwild.com

Monterey Bay Aquarium Seafood Watch: Sustainable seafood options
SeafoodWatch.org

Slow Food: International organization working to preserve traditional foods
slowfood.com

the kitchn: Answers to all your culinary questions and conundrums
thekitchn.com

The World's Healthiest Foods: Nutrients guide and health food information
whfoods.com

US Department of Agriculture: National Nutrient Database for Standard Reference
ndb.nal.usda.gov

BOOKS AND RESEARCH MATERIALS

The following is a list of sources consulted during the writing of this book.

Books

Colbin, Annemarie. *Food and Healing*. New York: Random House, 1986.

_____. *The Whole-Food Guide to Strong Bones*. Oakland, CA: New Harbinger Publications, 2009.

Enig, Mary. *Know Your Fats: The Complete Primer for Understanding the Nutrition of Fats, Oils and Cholesterol*. Silver Spring, MD: Bethesda Press, 2000.

Fallon, Sally. *Nourishing Traditions*. Washington, DC: NewTrends Publishing, 2001.

Katz, Rebecca. *The Longevity Kitchen*. Berkeley, CA: Ten Speed Press, 2013.

Kresser, Chris. *The Paleo Cure*. New York: Little Brown and Company, 2014.

Medrich, Alice. *Flavor Flours*. New York: Artisan, 2014.

Morgan, Diane. *Roots: The Definitive Compendium with More Than 225 Recipes*. San Francisco: Chronicle Books, 2012.

Pollan, Michael. *In Defense of Food: An Eater's Manifesto*. New York: Penguin Books, 2009.

_____. *The Omnivore's Dilemma*. New York: Penguin Books, 2007.

Schmid, Ronald. *Traditional Foods Are Your Best Medicine*. Rochester, VT: Healing Arts Press, 1997.

Speck, Maria. *Simply Ancient Grains*. Berkeley, CA: Ten Speed Press, 2015.

Wood, Rebecca. *The New Whole Foods Encyclopedia*. New York: Penguin Group, 2010.

Articles, Research, and Web Sites

American College of Sports Medicine, American Dietetic Association, and Dietitians of Canada. "Joint Position Statement: Nutrition and Athletic Performance." *Medicine and Science in Sports and Exercise* 32, no. 12 (December 2000): 2130–45.

Burns, Sarah. "Nutritional Value of Fruits, Veggies Is Dwindling." *NBC News*, July 9, 2010.

Centers for Disease Control and Prevention. "Chronic Disease Overview." Last updated January 20, 2016. cdc.gov/chronicdisease/overview.

Couric, Katie, Laurie David, and Stephanie Soechtig. *Fed Up*. fedupmovie.com.

Gerlach, K. E., et al. "Fat Intake and Injury in Female Runners." *Journal of the International Society of Sports Nutrition* 5, no. 1 (January 3, 2008).

Gordon, Elaine. "Teff, Ethiopia's Nutritious Grain." *Washington Post*, April 8, 2014.

Lim, S. S., et al. "A Comparative Risk Assessment of Burden of Disease and Injury Attributable to 67 Risk Factors and Risk Factor Clusters in 21 Regions, 1990-2010: A Systematic Analysis for the Global Burden of Disease Study 2010." *Lancet* 380, no. 9859 (December 25, 2012): 2224–60.

Lucas, L., A. Russel, and R. Keast. "Molecular Mechanisms of Inflammation. Anti-Inflammatory Benefits of Virgin Olive Oil and the Phenolic Compound Oleocanthal." *Current Pharmaceutical Design* 17, no. 8 (2011): 754–68.

Mahapatra, Lisa. "The US Spends Less on Food Than Any Other Country in the World." *International Business Times*, January 23, 2014.

Mallinson, R., et al. "A Case Report of Recovery of Menstrual Function following a Nutritional Intervention in Two Exercising Women with Amenorrhea of Varying Duration." *Journal of the International Society of Sports Nutrition* 10 (August 2, 2013): 34.

Mattes, R. D., P. M. Kris-Etherton, and G. D. Foster. "Impact of Peanuts and Tree Nuts on Body Weight and Healthy Weight Loss in Adults." *Journal of Nutrition* 138, no. S9 (September 2008): S1741–S1745.

Murphy, M., et al. "Whole Beetroot Consumption Acutely Improves Running Performance." *Journal of the Academy of Nutrition and Dietetics* 112, no. 4 (April 2012): 548–52.

Olshansky, J., et al. "A Potential Decline in Life Expectancy in the United States in the 21st Century." *New England Journal of Medicine* 352, no. 11 (March 17, 2005): 1138–45.

Roupas, N. D., and N. A. Georgopoulos. "Menstrual Function in Sports." *Hormones* 10, no. 2 (April-June 2011): 104–16.

Thompson, A. K., A. M. Minihane, and C. M. Williams. "Trans Fatty Acids and Weight Gain." *International Journal of Obesity* 35, no. 3 (March 2011): 315–24.

Warren, Michelle P. "Health Issues for Women Athletes: Exercise-Induced Amenorrhea." *Journal of Clinical Endocrinology and Metabolism* 84, no. 6 (June 1999): 1892–96.

Willett, W. C., and R. L. Leibel. "Dietary Fat Is not a Major Determinant of Body Fat." *American Journal of Medicine* 113 no. S9B (December 30, 2002): S47–S59.

Williams, N. I., et al. "Evidence for a Causal Role of Low Energy Availability in the Induction of Menstrual Cycle Disturbances during Strenuous Exercise Training." *Journal of Clinical Endocrinology and Metabolism* 86, no. 11 (November 2001): 5184–93.

World Health Organization. "Noncommunicable Diseases." Fact sheet, updated January 2015. www.who.int/mediacentre/factsheets/fs355/en/.

ACKNOWLEDGMENTS

This book would not be possible without the love and support from countless friends, family, and fans. Together we would like to express our sincerest gratitude to:

The hardworking team at Rodale books, including Aly Mostel, Evan Klonsky, Chris Gaugler, Jeff Batzli, Nancy N. Bailey, Susan Hindman, Anna Cooperberg, and our editor and chief liaison every step of the way, Dervla Kelly.

Our agent, Danielle Svetcov, for being our guiding light, supporting our endless drive, believing in this book from day one, and answering silly questions every step of the way.

Alan Weiner, our talented and extremely hardworking photographer, and Ashley Marti, our incredible food stylist. Thanks for making our book more beautiful than we ever imagined.

Our loyal cookbook assistant, Natalie Bickford, for her nutrition expertise, talent in the kitchen, and willingness to bounce between helping with the book, Lily, and Huck. You have a bright and rewarding career ahead of you.

Our friends and talented design visionaries, Tad Greenough and Sezay Altinok. Thank you for cooking up the brilliant idea for our cover.

Chef Cathy Whims, Doctor JJ Pursell, Tressa Yellig, Christine Mineart, Natalie Bickford, and Rebecca Katz, for contributing delicious recipes and guidance.

Megan Scott, from the *Joy of Cooking*, for professionally testing every single recipe, and John Becker, for professionally tasting every single recipe.

Draper Girls Country Farm, for welcoming us onto your gorgeous farm to photograph the outdoor shots in our book.

Our team of dedicated recipe testers with serious skills on the road and in the kitchen: Matt Llano, Amy Comander, Olivia Castellini, Ariel Tindolph, John Paul Robb, Amy Wolff, Sara Daum, Nikki Zielinski, Ashley Crossman, Maureen Atkins, Kim McDevitt, Clarissa Whiting, and Pam Hess.

And a special shout-out to our friends who volunteered to test recipes in their early stages: Jennie DiGiovanna, Maggie Flanagan, Emily Infeld, Cheryl Treworgy, Jane Finck, Brittany Williams, Danielle Quatrochi, Jessa Lyders, Margo Marver, Lydia Gaylord, Topher Gaylord, Michelle Gilpin, Megan Hetzel, Elliott Heath, Hayley Ney, and Chris Derrick.

SHALANE THANKS

My hearts swells with gratitude to the following people:

My parents, Monica and Steve Flanagan and Cheryl Treworgy, for your love and support and for teaching a shy little girl at a young age to "dare to be different."

My husband, Steve Edwards, for always supporting my passions. You encouraged Elyse and me to take a running leap into the unknown and believed in our book every step of the way.

Brother and sister, John Stephen and Maggie, for always daring to dream along with me.

Shubie, my sweet kitty, for your endless entertainment in the kitchen, while I tested and devoured every recipe in this book.

Bowerman Track Club teammates, for your

willingness to be our guinea pigs and test out our recipes on your road to Rio. You inspire me every day with your determination, perseverance, and dedication. I am grateful for your contagious smiles, laughs, and stories.

Nike Running, for seeing potential in me when I was fresh out of school and for supporting my athletic dreams for the past 12 years.

The Boston Athletic Association, John Hancock, and New York Road Runners, for giving me the platform to challenge myself against the best in the world.

My dedicated coaches, Jerry Schumacher and Pascal Dobert, for allowing a woman to join your team of men and letting me stay. Your unwavering commitment fuels my love for what I do.

Elyse Kopecky, my dearest friend of 16 years, for having the courage to pursue our wildest dream, for creating a list in college of things you wanted to accomplish, and then proceeding to check them off—talk about inspiration! Thank you for always following your heart and living with intention, and last but not least, for enhancing my kitchen skills! I'm so lucky to be on this joyful journey with you.

ELYSE THANKS

This dream became a reality thanks to a loyal cheering squad:

Shalanagan, for being an incredible friend and inspiration for over 16 years. You motivated me to pour the same drive into our book that you pour into your training and convinced me to take the plunge and follow my passion. You never blinked an eye at my obsessing over every detail, my spreadsheets, and my endless text messages. Even after a grueling 20-mile training run, you were always willing to jump into the kitchen. It's been a "phenomenal" journey and I could not have asked for a better co-author. Lily is so lucky to have you as an aunty to look up to (thanks for letting her teethe on your Olympic medal!).

Sissie Jessa Lyders, for teaching me to strive for perfection, for embracing this project wholeheartedly, and for being a big part of the inspiring story behind this book.

Lil bro Todd Kopecky, for your encouragement, enthusiasm, and dedication to reading and editing every word I've ever written. Thanks for the many grammar lessons over the phone. "When the sun comes up, you better be running . . . or writing."

Mom, Caren Arlas, for making this book possible by moving across country to take care of Lily so I could meet every deadline. I see the same appetite for learning in Lily that you inspired in me.

In loving memory of my dad, Ray Kopecky, for bringing home the first nutrition book I ever read (Dr Weil's *Spontaneous Healing*) and for underlining every passage that would help my running career. I still have the book and will forever treasure the notes you left for me within each chapter.

My oldest friend, Jane Finck, for inviting me into your home in NYC so that I could study at Natural Gourmet Institute. This dream would not have been possible without yours and Greg's generosity.

Diane Morgan, for your inspiring food writing class, your mentorship and friendship, and your dedication to Portland Culinary Alliance.

Friend and mentor, Kate Delhagen, for your guidance and belief in this project since its infancy.

The team of incredibly talented people at Nike Running that I had the honor of working alongside and learning from for 10 years.

Darya Rose, for believing in my recipes when I was fresh out of culinary school and for sending me the largest stack of books on how to write a book proposal.

The talented chefs at the Natural Gourmet Institute, for teaching me how to transform healthy food into indulgent dishes.

Coach Gil Murdock, you will never be forgotten. You inspired a lifelong passion for running by inviting me to join your XC team when I was a scrawny 12-year-old.

Belle-mère, Laurence Hughes, for your French influence on my culinary style, for teaching me how to make the best quiche crust, and for your love and support.

Lily, for spending more time in the kitchen in your first year of life than most kids spend in a lifetime. Seeing you devour my nourishing recipes with adorable enthusiasm brings me endless joy.

And last but certainly not least, my husband, Andy Hughes, for your love and support every step of the way, for making it possible for me to take this plunge, for always being up for a big adventure, and for being the most loyal dishwasher.

ABOUT THE AUTHORS

SHALANE FLANAGAN is an Olympic medalist, four-time Olympian, American record holder, and world-class marathoner. She finished second at the 2010 NYC marathon and ran the fastest time ever by an American woman at the 2014 Boston Marathon, completing the race in 2:22.02. At the 2014 Berlin Marathon, Shalane ran a personal best of 2:21.14, the second-fastest time ever by an American woman.

Nike has sponsored Shalane since she graduated from the University of North Carolina at Chapel Hill in 2004. She has been running at an elite level for 16 years and typically runs 100-plus miles a week. She attributes her ability to sustain this level of training to her nutrient-dense diet. Focusing on fueling for health and performance is an integral part of her training regimen.

Shalane has been featured on the cover of *Runner's World, Women's Running, Running Times, Competitor Magazine,* and *Track and Field News*. She has appeared on *60 Minutes, ESPN Outside the Lines,* and *Oprah*. Her inspiring story has also been heralded in *Women's Health, Shape, USA Today*, the *Boston Globe,* and the *New York Times*. Shalane speaks passionately about the importance of healthy eating at running events across the country. She lives and trains in Portland, Oregon.

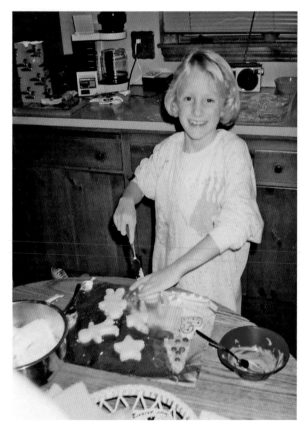

Shalane baking cookies at her grandma's house in 1988.

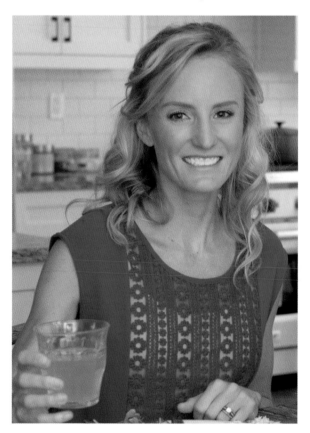

ELYSE KOPECKY is a chef, food writer, nutrition educator, runner, and proud mother. Her friendship with Shalane began 16 years ago on the cross-country team at the University of North Carolina. After graduation, both moved to Portland, Oregon, to work for Nike—Shalane as a professional runner, and Elyse as a digital marketing producer.

Elyse's career took her abroad, where she took cooking classes throughout Europe, Africa, and Asia. Armed with amazing recipes from around the world, Elyse began cooking to fuel her athletic endeavors. She discovered that by incorporating more fats into her diet, she was stronger, healthier, and happier than ever before. She quit a successful marketing career of 10 years for the chance to help others eat right and moved to New York City to study at the Natural Gourmet Institute for Health and Culinary Arts.

Once back in Portland, Elyse reunited with Shalane over a home-cooked meal, and their conversation quickly shifted to the detrimental fad diets pushed on female athletes. Elyse's infectious enthusiasm for teaching other women the importance of "indulgent nourishment" inspired Shalane. That night, the idea for *Run Fast Eat Slow* was born between two friends with a shared passion to educate and coach athletes to nourish themselves for the long run.

Find Elyse at IndulgentNourishment.com and on the trails in Bend, Oregon.

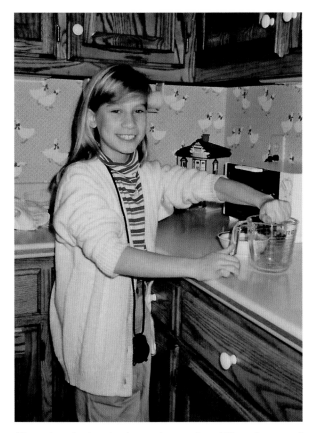

Elyse already showing her recipe-testing skills at the age of 11 (note the running stopwatch).

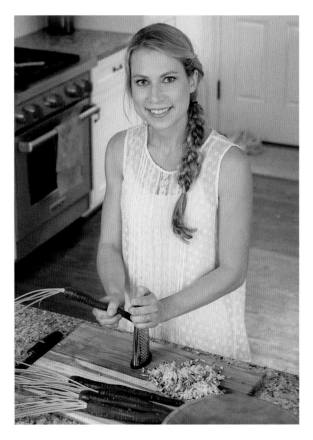

INDEX